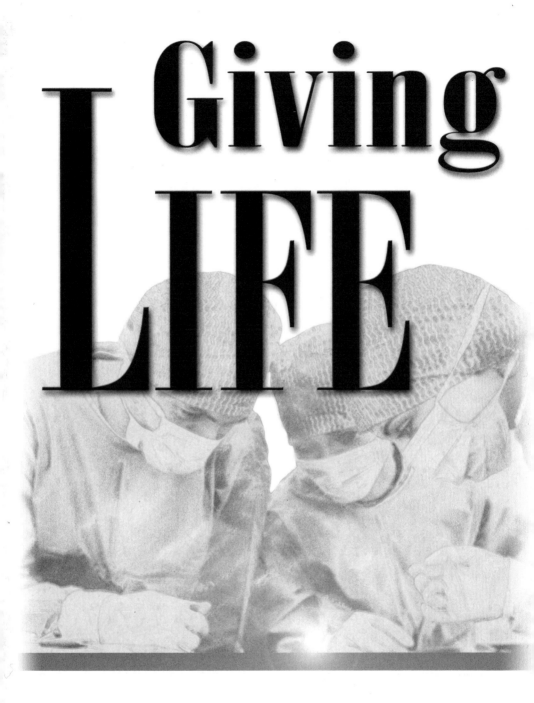

Giving LIFE

Inspirational Stories of Hope for Organ Donors and Recipients

by Tom Falsey

Copyright © 2008 Crystal Vision Books
P.O. Box 3185
Shawnee, Kansas 66216

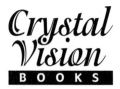

Written and Edited by Tom Falsey

First Edition

ISBN-13: 978-0-9795496-1-8
ISBN-10: 0-9795496-1-2

This publication is designed to provide accurate and authoritative information in regard to the subject matter covered. It is sold with the understanding that the publisher is not engaged in rendering legal, accounting, or other professional services. If legal advice or other expert assistance is required, the services of a competent professional should be sought.

Dedication

This book is dedicated to organ and tissue donors, both living and deceased.

To living donors who have made the courageous decision to donate a kidney, or piece of liver, lung, pancreas or intestine. Although long-term risks to donors are not well known, they have put their own health aside to help others in need.

To deceased donors and their families, who have given others renewed life when their own life has been cut short. Some deceased donors made their wishes known ahead of time giving family comfort in a time of unimaginable pain. Others left the decision to family members, and yet the gift is just as precious.

Table of Contents

Introduction vii

1   Take My Kidney – Please 1

2   Lyric's Light Shines On Through Others 9

3   A Survivor Helps Her Father 15

4   A Simple Matter Of Stewardship 23

5   Bronze-Medal Performance Gold-Medal Story 31

6   A Gigantic Assist 41

7   Allyson Gets A Great Deal 49

8   Fox News Correspondent's Living Donor
     Transplant Saved Her Infant Son 55

9   A Child's Legacy of Love 61

10 Brian Gets His Second Wind 67

11 Relief At Last 77

12 The Redford Family's Private Crisis 85

13 A Shared Kidney 93

14 No Way I Wouldn't Help 101

15 He Saved Her Life, She Saved His 107

16 Where Is Father Pat's Kidney? 113

17 Making The Right Choice – Twice 123

18 You Taught Me About Love 129

19 Lili Keeps On Blooming 135

20 A Gift For Mario 145

21 A Test Of Faith In Strangers 165

22 Losing A Kidney, Gaining A Family 179

23 Why Wouldn't She? 187

24 Meeting My 'Angel' 199

25 Here's Looking At You Kidney 205

26 Caring For Kari 215

27 A Life With Kidney Problems 231

27 A Gift Given – And Received 247

28 I Never Asked The Question 253

Epilogue 261

Organ Donation & Religion 265

Introduction

Miracles Happen

Miracles happen. They happen every single day and are, in fact, so commonplace that we do not always think of them as miracles. But for those whose lives have been touched by those miracles, it is impossible to deny they exist.

What I am referring to is the miracle of organ transplantation. Organ transplantation has only been in existence for a little more than fifty years. From the time the first kidney was successfully transplanted in 1954, thousands and thousands of people have benefited from the "Gift of Life," a life extended or improved because someone was kind enough to donate an organ. Literally hundreds of thousands of people have received this gift. On an average day more than seventy people receive a life saving organ transplant in the United States. Unfortunately, on that same day, about 18 people will die because no organ is available.

Think a moment about what organ donation is. A skilled surgeon can take the heart of a dead person and give it to a sick person, who then becomes healthy. Another surgeon can split the liver of a living donor, giving part of it to a person with liver disease. Both the donor and recipient have a healthy liver that grows back to its original size.

Transplantation has become so common place that it may not be considered a miracle. Tell that to a person whose life has been freed from dialysis because of a kidney transplant. Or to a mother of an infant who just received a new heart. Or to the father who lost his own child in an automobile accident, and gets to feel his child's heart beat in someone else's chest.

I consider myself lucky because I have seen the miracle of transplantation several times. I have had the joy of seeing its successful outcome. And what is more, I have seen it happen over and over again.

My first experience with organ transplantation occurred in 1990, when my nephew Aaron received a kidney donated by his mother. Aaron had been so sick as a teenager suffering from kidney disease, and then he received a transplant. He went from a small sickly child to a healthy young man in a very short period of time. And his mother, his kidney donor? Yes, she hurt quite badly and her recovery was slow. The surgery was harder back then, but she recovered nicely and no longer remembers the pain.

Several years later, Aaron's kidney failed and he needed a second transplant. He had rejected his mother's transplanted kidney and had it surgically removed in preparation for a second transplant. It was not meant to be however, the surgery was called off two days before it was scheduled to take place. He and his donor had a positive cross-match – a sign that he would reject this kidney too. There was no point in going forward.

Aaron refused to accept another kidney donation from a family member, preferring not to put anyone through that pain again. He would rather die than see someone he loved make that sacrifice – and he almost did. A delivery man who inexplicably knew something was wrong when he tried to drop off his dialysis solution saved his life. His persistence in ringing the doorbell was enough to awaken Aaron from a near coma as he had fallen asleep two days earlier, and had not awakened since. Once awakened, Aaron was able to make it to the hospital for help.

Although Aaron did not want a kidney from a family member, his sister Michelle had other ideas. She got tested without his knowledge and learned she was a match. Aaron had seen his determined sister before when she made up her mind to do something, and knew he had virtually no choice. He graciously accepted her kidney donation in 2002 and both he and Michelle are doing just fine.

My third experience with organ donation happened in July of 2003 and touched me even more personally. At The Nebraska Medical Center in Omaha, I became the first donor to anonymously donate a kidney. I did not know who the recipient would be, but I was wheeled into an operating room and gave up my left kidney. I knew I had two and someone else needed one. As it turned out, the kidney went to a teenaged boy much like Aaron who had lost his kidney function.

I learned a little about sibling rivalry the following year when my older brother, Jim, decided to follow suit. He donated a kidney anonymously at St. John's hospital in Detroit, giving his kidney to a thirty-nine year-old woman named, Karen. That is all he knew about her, except that he knew she was sick and that he could help.

Our family and its stories of kidney donation were not yet complete. Before Jim had his surgery, my wife Joyce decided she could do it too. Later that same year she donated her kidney anonymously. Her kidney went to Regina, an African American woman who had lost her kidney function due to Lupus.

Having five kidney donors in one family is unusual, but it is not heroic. Our family has seen the miracle of organ donation take place over and over again. For us to have been lucky enough to take part in this miracle, we are indeed blessed.

I have never met an organ donor who considers himself or herself a hero. It is more of a calling. Although it is not for everyone, for those who choose it, the rewards can be great.

The purpose of this book is not to convince you or anyone else to become an organ donor. Rather, it is to have you think about organ donation, and hopefully you will learn that this miracle is something you can become a part of if you choose to do so.

Organs for transplantation come from two sources, living donors and deceased donors. Stories told here involve both types of donors. Each donor has given another person an opportunity of a better life.

Living donors have the opportunity to see what the "gift of life" means to someone else. Deceased donors will never get to experience that feeling. The gift of life is just that – it is a gift, and it gives life. It really is that simple.

I like to say that donating a kidney is the most significant thing that I have done in my life, but that does not make me a hero. The real heroes are the doctors and surgeons who can remove an organ from one body (living or deceased) and install it in another where it will keep the beat of life going. It is a miracle that was simply a dream more than fifty years ago and is now commonplace. Chances are you know of someone who has experienced an organ transplant. Many of those simply would not be alive today if it were not for organ donation.

I should point out that no one wants you to become a deceased organ donor. Organ donation is not about death, it is about life. We truly want everyone to live healthy lives. But death does happen, and it will happen to all of us someday. Most of us will not be eligible to become deceased organ donors*. We will live full lives and die at an old age when our organs are no longer of any use to a person in need. But challenge yourself to think about what you would want to happen if you are one of the unlucky ones who dies young, and in certain circumstances.

If you should become brain-dead, what would you want to happen? Unfortunately, if that happens to you, it is too late to decide – you are already dead. If you have signed the back of your driver's license or signed up on the donor registry, that may not be enough. In many states, it is not up to you, it is up to your family, and your family will be facing some very tough decisions if put in this situation. The last thing they will want to do is to make a mistake. The only way they can honor your decision is if they know your wishes. That knowledge needs to be shared while you are alive.

Talk to your family and let them know what you think about organ and tissue donation.

*Never assume that you are too old to be a donor. Organs and tissue come from donors of all ages – you are never too young or old to be a donor.

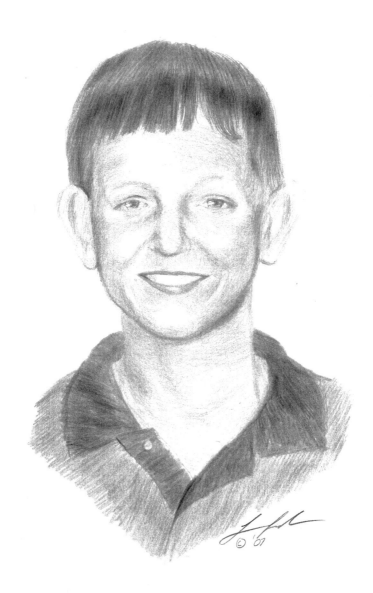

**Jordan Shaw
Kidney Recipient**

Take My Kidney – Please

I met Jordan Shaw in November 2003. Sixteen years old and small for his age, Jordan stood only about four feet eleven inches tall and weighed barely 85 pounds. Jordan had had a hard time in life, harder than most people experience in a lifetime. In spite of his poor health, though, he was one of the friendliest people I have had the pleasure of meeting.

When he was two years old, Jordan was diagnosed with a rare form of cancer that required him to undergo chemotherapy. The chemotherapy worked on his cancer, but damaged his urinary system. His kidneys grew weaker as the years progressed and eventually ceased functioning altogether.

Jordan was on dialysis that kept him alive, but it was not the kind of life you'd expect or hope for a teenager. Jordan had to get up early each morning to be at the dialysis center by 5:30 a.m. When he got home from school, he often went straight to bed, too tired to do anything else.

Jordan missed 43 days of school in 2002-2003 and had to attend summer school to make up for the time he had missed. He was alive, but what kind of life did he have?

In July 2003, Jordan received a kidney transplant that made a world of difference in him. The color returned to his face immediately. The change was so dramatic that he could see his own freckles for the first time in years. Prior to that, he had been so pale the freckles simply didn't show. He had even forgotten he had freckles until his health returned.

He no longer needed the dialysis to stay alive and no longer needed to get up so early. He could watch television late into the night because he was no longer tired. Once his mother came downstairs to make her morning coffee, only to find Jordan playing video games. He felt so good that he didn't realize it was six o'clock in the morning. He had played games all night.

It was a pleasure to meet Jordan because we had a shared bond. Although we had never met before that November day, we had something in common.

Jordan was the first to receive a kidney transplant in an innovative program at The Nebraska Medical Center, and I was his donor. The kidney that was alive in me for 48 years was now making a difference in Jordan's life. Although his new kidney was older than both of his parents, that didn't matter to him. It was his 'new kidney' now.

Four months had passed since the transplant, and we met for the first time. In those four months we had wondered about each other. Each of us wanted to know more about the other.

It was ironic that our meeting took place two days

after a much-promoted interstate football game between Kansas State and Nebraska. I live in Kansas, and Jordan lives in Nebraska. The rivalry between the two schools meant nothing when it comes to organ transplants, however. Jordan didn't care where the kidney came from, and I didn't care where it went.

So what does this football game have in common with the kidney Jordan and I share? Not much, really, except that the game was played at Cornhusker stadium in Lincoln, Nebraska, and, even though the stadium holds more than 80,000 people, it still is not big enough to hold all of those on the waiting list for organ transplants. And the number of those in need continues to grow each day.

There are two ways to get off the waiting list — either to get a transplant or to become too sick to be transplanted. The first is a miracle of modern medicine; the other is a tragedy of a life wasted. The first is an opportunity to help a person live; the other is the result of no help being offered.

The Anonymous Donor Program at The Nebraska Medical Center and other programs like it are designed to help empty the stadium, one person at a time. It helps people with few options get off the waiting list and get back into the game of life.

Who are the people that need organ transplants? There's no easy category into which all of these individuals fit. There are people like Jordan, who got cancer at a young age. There are people who destroyed their organs because they did not take care of themselves. Others, born prematurely, have organs that did not develop properly. Still others simply encountered health problems that destroyed their organs.

Organ failure can happen to anyone, even the rich and famous. Walter Payton and Barry White died waiting for organ transplants. Larry Hagman had a liver transplant and lived. Mickey Mantle had a liver transplant and died.

How nice would it have been to save Walter Payton's life? Or Barry White's? How fulfilling would it be to donate part of a liver to Larry Hagman to enhance his life? Or to donate it to Mickey Mantle even though it only extended his life by a month?

Robert Redford's son Jamie has had two liver transplants. The first transplant was unsuccessful; the liver failed right away. The second transplanted liver, however, saved his life.

Anonymous donor programs are designed to match willing donors with needy patients who have few options. A transplant means there is one less person on the waiting list.

So many people are in need of a life-saving transplant that the goal may seem hopeless. No one can help them all, but many can help one. One by one, people can move off the list because of a transplanted organ. The organ may come from a deceased donor–a person tragically killed in an automobile accident or similar tragedy; it can come from a living person – a relative or friend who took the time to be tested; or, it can come from an anonymous donor; a stranger who just wants to make a difference in someone's life.

What would compel someone to become a living donor? Isn't that a serious operation? Aren't there risks?

Yes, it is a serious operation and there certainly are risks to the donor, but for me, the rewards outweigh the risks. I know from my own personal experience that the rewards are great.

To be a donor, you have to be healthy. The tests are extensive. Some potential donors have gone through the testing only to find a problem that prevents them from donating. Finding the problem early is always better than finding it late. Imagine trying to save someone else's life and ending up saving your own.

The most dramatic thing to me was the prayer offered in my name. A kidney transplant is serious surgery, and not without risks. But with the risks come prayers. People who hear of your intention to donate pray for you. Friends, family, and even total strangers pray for you. Unsolicited prayer usually only happens when you are sick or dead, but I had people praying for me because I was healthy. I cannot tell you what that meant to me.

Tests had proven I had two healthy kidneys. Although I had one more than I needed, there were thousands of people who did not have any. Someone was going to get my 'extra' kidney.

I have often been asked what it was like to meet the person who had my 'old' kidney. Was it dramatic? How did I feel? What was it like? It was as if there should have been a miraculous 'Oprah Winfrey' moment where we both lost control of our emotions in a flood of tears. That would have been dramatic, but it simply was not like that.

What the moment lacked in a temporary burst of tears will be made up in time that follows. The joy I had at meeting Jordan pales in comparison to the joy of every day afterward. For I know that, today, Jordan will not be tied to a machine for four hours. Nor tomorrow. Nor the next day, or the day after that. Kidneys from living donors last 19 years on average and, for as long as mine lasts in him, he won't need dialysis.

Jordan is now allowed to live a life that teenagers are supposed to live. And, yes, he can cause problems and get into trouble now and again. He is young; that is his job. He can now do what he is supposed to do.

As for me? Physically, I am the same person I always was. I don't have to do anything different. The only differences are a few tiny scars I wear with pride. I take better care of myself, but I am getting older and I need to do that anyway.

Emotionally, I am different. The changes this has made in my life are numerous and difficult to describe. There is a satisfaction that no one can take away. This is certainly the best thing I ever did (and I slept through it).

I intended to enrich another life and ended up enriching my own. I have absolutely no regrets and would do it all over again if I had the chance.

Donating a kidney is not for everyone, but it was for me. It is the best move I've ever made. It wasn't done for selfish reasons, but I've gained more than I have lost. I have gained more than I could possibly imagine.

The Wait List

Demand for transplantable organs is greater than the supply. Over the 10-year period from 1997 to 2006, the number of people on the wait list for organs has nearly doubled (from 53,167 to 94,441). During the same time, the number of organs transplanted has grown less than 50 percent (from 20,307 to 28,931).

As soon as the numbers are posted, they become outdated. In 2006 (the last full year with data available), a new name was added to the list every 11 seconds. Each day more than 18 people on the list died because no organ was available.

Transplants Performed vs. the Wait List

The chart below shows the number of transplants performed annually and the number of people on the wait list at the end of the year.

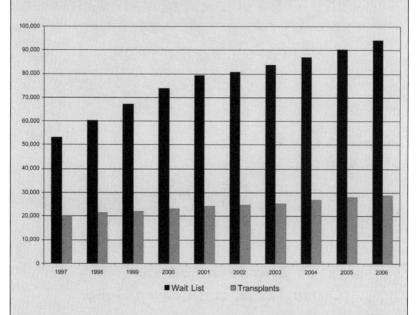

Based on OPTN/UNOS data as of May 24, 2007

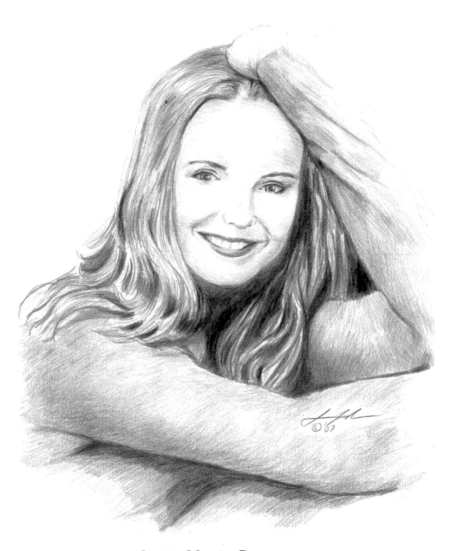

Lyric Marie Benson
Organ, Tissue, and Cornea Donor

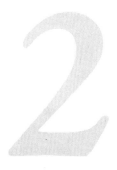

Lyric's Light Shines On Through Others

By Terry Benson (Lyric's Father)

Just after midnight on September 20, 1980, a beautiful blessing occurred. Lyric.

Suburban Hospital in Overland Park, Kansas, was illuminated that day as Lyric Marie Benson began a wonderful journey through which she captured the hearts and souls of those she touched along the way.

I'm often asked how Lyric was named. I remember well being on the way to the Lyric Theater with Lyric's mom, Deborah, who was about eight months pregnant. Going through name games was fun, but it had not really gotten us anywhere. We wanted something unique, but not too bizarre.

Because the Lyric Theater was our destination, I suddenly said, "What about Lyric?" Instead of offering the usual reasons for not accepting a name, Deborah was silent. That turned out to be a good sign. Lyric inherited her middle name from my mother, Wynona Marie Mihura.

A child who immediately began 'soaking in' the world, Lyric favored learning and reading over tantrums and tirades. An early and avid reader, she was rarely found without several books accompanying her.

Lyric helped balance her childhood with efforts in athletics. From about age seven through high school, she participated in soccer, basketball, track, volleyball, and softball. Though she knew that sports were not her destiny, she developed textbook techniques shooting a basketball, and throwing or batting a softball.

Her love for life seemed to have followed her poetic name. Lyric began to develop a "sense of the dramatic" at an early age. She was funny, clever, creative, expressive, and engaging with family and friends. It was at age six, however, that she first performed at a deck party in front of many people. With the evening's theme being lip-sync, Lyric captivated everyone with three songs. She was the unexpected star of the party!

After that night, there were more than 10 lip-sync deck parties in which Lyric wowed the crowd. During those years, she learned to play the piano, and the violin, and developed a true singing talent. Attending and performing in theater became her desire. Entertaining was a part of her.

After attending her prep years at an American school in Casablanca, Morocco, Lyric was prepared for the biggest and best parts of her life. Having graduated as valedictorian of her high school, she was selected to attend Yale, where she graduated in Theater Studies, with honors. Her next step was the Big Apple.

Within a few months, Lyric was working hard through her casting agents to compete in a tough industry. With her evening work as a hostess at a popular restaurant, and routine dedication in the gym, she was becoming a part of her New York surroundings. Auditions began to click. She earned minor roles with *Comedy Central, All My Children*, and *Law and Order*, and did commercial voice-overs.

Her biggest breakthrough came with a print ad in the *New Yorker* magazine for American Express, sponsor of the TriBeCa Film Festival. That ad blossomed into numerous posters and billboards throughout New York City. She was on her way.

Then, the unimaginable. In April 2003, Lyric was tragically gunned down at close range in New York City by an ex-boyfriend. Getting the news at 3 a.m. was stunning! Unbelievable! Horrific! A nightmare! How could this possibly be true? It was nearly impossible to assimilate. As the family scrambled to be by her side at Bellevue Hospital, there was an obvious choice to make.

Deborah, a teacher, had previously witnessed the miracle of life in her own second-grade classroom in Beaufort, North Carolina. The sadness of watching a young boy slipping away from heart disease turned to happiness due to a life-saving heart transplant. That was a good reason for Lyric to discuss becoming a donor. It would become her final fate.

Her love for life transcended this extremely dark moment for us into brighter ones for others. Her organ and tissue donation saved five lives, offered the opportunity for further life-enhancing surgeries, and helped with research. As much as this was the end of a beautiful life, Lyric's legacy continued to unfold through a nonprofit association called *LYRIC of LIFE*.

From support of generous people who knew and loved Lyric, along with many who have come to know her, *LYRIC of LIFE* has begun a journey of helping others. *LOL* brings awareness to the need for organ donation, directly helps donor and recipient families with short-term financial assistance, and grants theater scholarships to high-school seniors who closely emulate what Lyric stood for.

LOL benefits have been held in April, the month of Lyric's life-saving organ donations, each year since 2004. The event champions Lyric's creative and beautiful years, and her world travels. She now symbolizes the essence of success in how she maintained a humble stature, kept family close to her heart, lived to learn, maintained a spiritual peace, and reached for limitless dreams.

Lyric was a beautiful person in all ways. Her light now shines on through others. Her memory is a blessing etched forever in our minds. She loved life. She gave life.

LYRIC of LIFE
P.O. BOX 4142
Overland Park, Kansas 66204

www.LYRICofLIFE.org

To Become a Donor

If you want to become an organ or tissue donor at the time of your death, it is important to make your wishes known. Your family may be asked to make a very difficult decision, and that decision will be far easier if they know what you would want to do. The best way to assure your wishes are honored is to make them known.

To document your decision on organ and tissue donation at your death:

1. **Join your state donor registry.** You can obtain information on joining the donor registry in your state by visiting www.donatelife.net.

2. **Designate your decision on your driver's license.** You can do this when you obtain or renew your driver's license.

3. **Sign a donor card.** At www.organdonor.gov, you can download an organ donation card to carry with you.

4. **Talk with your family.** The most important thing you can do is to talk with your family. Let them know what your wishes are. If they have to make the decision for you, it is too late for them to ask.

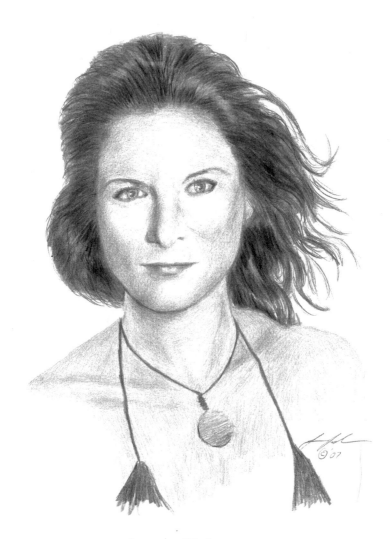

**Leann Slaby
Kidney Donor**

3

A Survivor Helps Her Father
by Leann Slaby

After the birth of my sister and brother, my parents were told that they could not have any more children. Wanting another child, and determined to prove the doctors wrong, my parents tried to conceive again. To their delight, I was born on July 8, 1969...and my parents called me their "miracle baby."

Maybe there's a reason for such things. Maybe I was given the gift of life so that I could return the favor someday.

My father was diagnosed with diabetes when he was 16. Experts were fairly sure that he developed the disease as a result of a hunting accident in which he was shot in the abdominal area. For 38 years, my father lived with Type 1 diabetes without any kidney problems. However, in late 1997 we learned that his kidneys were failing.

I come from a very close family. We've suffered through the years from many of the same tribulations that other families do, and probably more. But every obstacle or problem that arose for our tight-knit family always resulted in strengthened relationships and emotional closeness. This was no exception.

We all knew that the possibility was there... we knew there were a number of things that could happen to diabetics. We just always hoped that Dad was the exception. I remember the day I first found out that Dad needed a kidney transplant. My immediate thought was that I was going to be the one to donate my kidney. I can't explain it. I just knew. Of course, going through the battery of tests to see if I was a match sparked anxiety – hoping that everything came back okay, and that I would be given the green light to donate – but deep down there was never a doubt that I would be his donor.

The whole family gathered at the University Hospital in Madison, Wisconsin, to meet with Dr. Hans Sollinger about kidney donation and what to expect. My siblings and my mother were all willing to be a donor for my dad, and would do it in a heartbeat. As much as we tried to convince him otherwise, I could tell that my father was uncomfortable with the prospect of putting someone he loved in harm's way for his benefit. But that's what families do... they sacrifice. At times they take, and at times they give. This was the one time where my father was to take, and it was up to us to give.

Support from the family came quickly and easily. My mother, my siblings Russ and Lisa, their spouses and I were all tested to see if we could be a potential match. Several of my father's siblings also were tested. While either of my siblings could have donated, as I suspected, I was the best match. Like I said, I just knew it. It seemed so right. My brother and my dad had a business together and it would have been hard on the business if they were both to be out of commission at the same time. My sister had a full-time job and a family at home. As for me, I had a job I could leave for an extended period of time and no kids at home. It was meant to be.

I went through a series of medical examinations and tests to make sure that I was fit to be a donor. It was pretty extensive and I was afraid of any little thing going wrong. But it turned out that I was in picture-perfect health.

The surgery was scheduled for March 5, 1998. I remember the day very clearly. Until that day, I had no worries. I felt no anxiety at all. But the morning of surgery I had a few moments of nervousness, mostly because my Mom and siblings were a little late getting to the hospital and I was afraid they would wheel me into surgery without the chance to talk to them!

It was such a medley of emotions. I worried about my Mom, who had both her husband and daughter in surgery at the same time. I worried about my Dad and prayed that he would handle the surgery well, but I think more than anything I was worried that it wouldn't work. I wanted so badly for the transplant to be successful. I didn't want my Dad to have to go through another surgery because my kidney wasn't good enough. I knew that, as wrong as it was, if the transplant had failed, both of us would have blamed ourselves.

I remember being put under anesthesia and singing Abba's "Take a Chance On Me" before I drifted off to sleep. I remember telling my friend Brenda, who was an ER nurse at the hospital and by my side as I was going under, "Don't let anyone see me naked." Funny.

As I came out of unconsciousness, I was told that the surgery was a success. Inside I felt elated, but I couldn't make my outsides do much yet. I did manage to ask where my Dad was. They told me that he was in the recovery room with me, across the room. I lifted my hundred-pound head and looked over at Dad. He did the same, and we both raised a weak arm in an attempt to communicate that everything is all right. It was a moment I'll never forget, and brings me to tears every time I think of it. There was something magical about that moment, despite how groggy I was.

That first night, the unyielding nurses had me up on my feet. I demanded that I go see my Dad. I was in a lot of pain, but it didn't matter. I baby stepped it over to my Dad's room where we held hands and shed a tear or 20. There was an unmistakable bond between us. It's something that I still can't explain, but it is undeniably there.

The days that followed were rough for both of us, but his numbers kept coming back good, and that's all that mattered. My father never rejected my kidney.

I find it funny that some people say it was "admirable" to have given my kidney to my father. I've always thought that *I* was the lucky one. How often does a child get the opportunity to give back the gift of life to one of the very people that gave that gift in the first place? I would do it over and over again, if I could.

In March 2007, we celebrated nine years of success with the transplant, and the kidney is still working wonderfully. Dad still e-mails or calls me with his creatinine results when he makes his follow-up visits. And it's always a sigh of relief when the numbers come back on target.

As for me, I still do the same things I've always

done, and I would never know that I only have one kidney. Aside from the surgery and the five weeks of recovery, there are no limitations on me physically. In fact, I've proven that a kidney donor can even do extraordinary things, like survive on a tropical island in the South Pacific for 30 days without the luxuries of home!

Early in 2004, I was chosen to be a contestant on CBS's *Survivor: Vanuatu,* which finished airing in December 2004. In my audition tape, I mentioned that I donated my kidney to my father and that part of the reason for my application was to show people that you can live an ordinary or even extraordinary life after becoming a living donor. My hope was to bring awareness to organ donation in general, since my father also received a pancreas transplant two years after the kidney transplant. Organ donation, living or otherwise, is a beautiful thing... a real gift that can truly enrich lives. I thought that going on the show and getting people talking about organ donation could only be a good thing. Unfortunately, the fact that I was a living donor never came out on the show itself!

Being on *Survivor* wasn't easy. For the first three days, we had no water. That was the only time that I was nervous about what effect this experience would have on my kidney. But on the third day, we won fire in a reward challenge, and were able to boil water to drink. Never once did I feel dehydrated, and my lone kidney came out unscathed! I think it's safe to assume that Mom and Dad's "miracle baby" came with some pretty heavy-duty kidneys, and they've served both me and Dad very well.

Dad never lets me forget how grateful he is, although he doesn't need to. If I could, I would give him my eye and my foot, too – both of which he lost to diabetes. Despite the difficulties he's endured from diabetes, he still leads a very normal, productive and active life, complete with an eternal positive attitude.

Our family celebrates each successful transplant year that goes by. We try to get together in March of each year for the annual kidney party. My sister Lisa has been in charge of the "kidney cake" (just like it sounds—a cake in the shape of a kidney!), and we gather together and essentially count our blessings. We're a pretty emotional family, so there are usually plenty of damp eyes in the house. And, if we can't seem to get together, I always get a little gift or note from Dad right around March 5, saying "thank you."

Unfortunately, the pancreas my father received in July 2000, from a young man who died suddenly, chronically rejected in early 2004. But for nearly four years, he was given the gift of a diabetes-free life, and may have also helped extend the life of his kidney.

No matter how you look at it, organ donation is an incredible gift. It can be a fulfilling offering to a loved one, or a beautiful way to give life after death.

Kidneys

The kidneys are a pair of reddish-brown organs located on either side of the spine just below the diaphragm, behind the liver and stomach. They are bean-shaped and about 4 and 1/2 inches long, 2 and 1/2 inches wide and one inch thick. The primary function of the kidneys is to remove waste from the body through the production of urine. They also help to regulate blood pressure, blood volume and the chemical (electrolyte) composition of the blood.

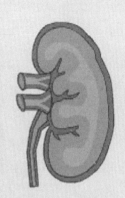

© United Network of Organ Sharing. Reprinted by permission.

U.S. Kidney Transplants Performed

The chart below shows the number of kidney transplants performed each year from 1997 to 2006.

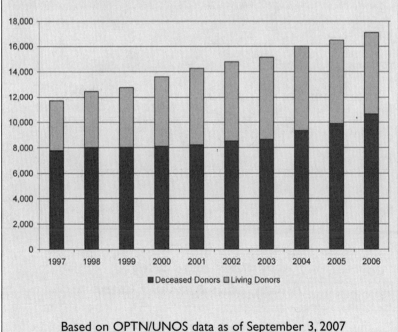

Based on OPTN/UNOS data as of September 3, 2007

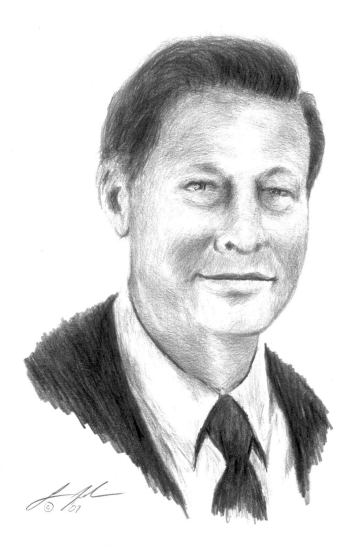

Father Jim Falsey
Anonymous Kidney Donor

4

A Simple Matter of Stewardship

As a Catholic priest, Father Jim Falsey believes in helping others in need. He often gives blood, thinking the cost of doing so is minimal, but the value is immense. It seems like such a small price to pay for something that could mean so much to a person in need. Fr. Jim leads his parish in Au Gres, Michigan, by example, often hosting blood drives for his parish. He has even challenged other churches in the area to see which church can collect the most blood.

During one of his blood donations, Fr. Jim was asked if he would be interested in signing up for the national bone marrow registry. By enrolling in the registry, the genetic make-up of his blood would be compared with people in need of a life-saving bone marrow transplant. Signing the registry would not obligate him to anything, but it could provide him the opportunity to save a life, should he be determined to be a match.

For some patients stricken with leukemia or lymphoma, a bone marrow transplant is their only opportunity for a cure. While some patients in need find genetic matches among family members, about 70 percent do not. Some have to rely on the kindness of strangers to become members of the bone marrow registry.

Fr. Jim asked a few questions about bone marrow donation and then figured, "Why not?" If he were to be a perfect match, he could save the life of someone in critical need. And he could do so with minimal risk to himself. There was no question this would be something he would like to do if he were to be fortunate enough to match.

Although Jim never found his perfect match for a bone marrow transplant, he took his mission one step further. After watching me, his youngest brother, donate a kidney anonymously, Fr. Jim decided he could consider doing the same thing.

My surgery moved Fr. Jim deeply, and after thinking about it for a while, he decided, "Hey, I could do that." He figured that, like the bone marrow registry, he would join the kidney donor registry, too. That way, he could donate a kidney if he matched a patient who needed one.

Jim contacted me to get more information. I had successfully donated a kidney and knew some of the ins and outs of the procedure. Jim wanted to talk with someone who had firsthand experience.

Although he was calling for advice, it was clear his mind was already made up. He started the conversation by simply stating, "If you can do it, I can do it, too."

At first I was hesitant. I had down played my kidney donation to the family because I did not want anyone to worry. But now my brother was considering making the same gift. Did he understand what he was saying? This is a big surgery and no one should take it lightly.

Although I had gone through the surgery with relative ease, I recognized I was one of the lucky ones. Would Jim have the same luck?

I was proud of my brother's decision and hopeful he would help another person get off the waiting list, but Jim had to make his own decision and he had to have the facts.

I had to let my brother know the truth: There is no kidney registry. Instead, there is a critical, ongoing need for kidneys, as well as other organs, and the need far exceeds the supply. It is not necessary that you be a perfect genetic match to be a donor. It is not even required that the donor and recipient are related. With anti-rejection drugs, virtually anyone who is healthy enough can be a donor. A genetic match is becoming less and less important.

About half the transplanted kidneys come from deceased donors, where there is rarely a biological relationship between the donor and recipient. In fact, the recipient rarely knows where the kidney came from. The other half of the kidneys transplanted come from living donors. Even with living donors, a biological relationship is becoming less important. More than a third of living donors are not biologically related to their recipients.

If you are willing to give up one of your kidneys, you will most likely match someone in need. All you have to do is prove that you are healthy enough to donate a kidney, that you are making a sane, informed decision, and that you are likely to have a normal life with only one kidney.

Fr. Jim considered kidney donation a matter of stewardship. "Stewardship begins with the basic principle that we do not 'own' anything. God 'owns' all that is." His words are backed up in the Bible, "The heavens, even the highest heavens, belong to the Lord, your God, as well as the earth and everything on it." (Deuteronomy 10:14)

Fr. Jim continues, "We are the stewards of God's creation. Everything we claim to possess is merely entrusted to us by God to be used in accord with His will for our good and the good of all His creatures. Not even our bodies belong exclusively to ourselves. Every mother who has given birth or nursed a child knows that."

After weighing the evidence, Fr. Jim gave this idea the careful consideration it deserved. He studied all the information he could find on organ donation and talked with others who were involved in this leading-edge medical field. And he prayed for guidance in making a decision that was right not only for himself, but also for someone else in need.

He came to the conclusion that he wanted to donate one of his healthy kidneys to someone he had never met. After all, he had two healthy kidneys and there was someone, somewhere, who did not have any. This was the right thing for him to do.

"I learned that the average person can live normally with only one kidney and still have plenty of kidney capacity to spare," Jim said.

Having arrived at a decision he was comfortable with, Fr. Jim had to find a place to donate his kidney. I had donated at The Nebraska Medical Center, but that would not work for Fr. Jim. He lived in Michigan and needed some place that was closer to home. He would have to go through several rounds of testing and the process would take months. He could not afford to travel back and forth to Nebraska.

With a little research on the Internet, Jim found two Michigan hospitals that might work for him. Both were about a three-hour drive from his home in Au Gres. Each hospital, St. John's Hospital and Medical Center in Detroit and the University of Michigan in Ann Arbor, had performed only one anonymous kidney donation.

He contacted both hospitals to learn about their programs. The staff at the University of Michigan was more experienced in kidney transplantation, but St. John's seemed to be more willing to work with an anonymous donor. After discussions with both transplant coordinators, he made his decision. Fr. Jim decided to pursue his dream of donating a kidney at St. John's.

With each round of testing, he was assured he had the right to change his mind. With each step forward, the staff tried to make sure he knew what he was doing and that he understood what his decision meant. This helped strengthen his resolve, making him even more certain this was the right thing for him to do. The entire process took several months and Fr. Jim passed each step with confidence.

In April 2004, the wait was over. Fr. Jim traveled to Detroit to give away his kidney. He did not know anything about his recipient, except her first name, Karen. The operation was scheduled for the week after Easter, so Fr. Jim brought an Easter card to give Karen along with his kidney. The card was passed through the transplant coordinator to make certain it was appropriate. Fr. Jim did not know Karen's faith and did not want to offend her.

Dr. Hawasli performed the laparoscopic surgery, taking Jim's left kidney. Fr. Jim became only the second anonymous kidney donor at St. John's Hospital and

Medical Center – and the second anonymous donor in the family.

Perhaps what is most unusual about his surgery was the ease of recovery. His recovery was somewhat longer than normal, but not because of complications. Fr. Jim was so comfortable and relaxed that he fell asleep in recovery and caught up on some much-needed rest.

After awaking from his nap, Jim was transferred to a semi-private room and hooked up to monitoring equipment that measured his vital statistics. There waiting for him were my wife, Joyce, and me. Both of us were amazed at how comfortable Jim appeared. Comparing his recovery to mine, I had thought I was one of the lucky ones because I didn't have any pain, but his surgeon made my surgeon look like an amateur.

Released from the hospital the day after surgery, Fr. Jim made the four-hour ride home with us without any problems. Along the way, we stopped only once to stretch and walk. The break was not for Jim's comfort; he was doing fine. The rest of us needed a bathroom break.

Within three days of surgery, Jim was back on the job celebrating Mass. Other than a slight stabbing pain when he raised the host in blessing, there was no noticeable difference detectable in the celebration. Most of his parishioners were not even aware that he had recently had major surgery. The few who did notice a difference were those in whom he had confided, hoping they would come to his rescue if he were pushing himself too far or too fast.

Since giving the gift of life, Fr. Jim has become an advocate for organ donation and shares his experience with others considering this act.

"I have been blessed with exceptionally good health.

If I could use part of my body to improve the quality of life for someone who is suffering, why not? That is what led me to donate a kidney. Some have called that 'heroic' or a 'great act.' No, not really. It is simply a matter of stewardship. I had two functioning kidneys, someone else had none. God had entrusted those kidneys to me. I believe I took good care of them; and they took good care of me. That left kidney had served me well for 59 years. Now it is someone else's responsibility. It is simply a matter of stewardship."

"Does that mean everyone should consider donating a kidney, a lung, part of their liver or some other body part? No, absolutely not! It does mean that we should carefully consider how we use, and care for, our bodies. They are not our own. They are not entrusted to us for ourselves alone. They are entrusted to us to be cared for and used in accord with God's will."

"For 99.9 percent of us, that means keeping our bodies intact. It means using them to make a decent living for ourselves, our families, and for the least of our brothers and sisters. It means using the time, the talents and the treasure that God has entrusted to us to build up the Kingdom of God. If, however, you find yourself thinking: 'I, too, have been exceptionally blessed. I could do that,' then give it some thought. Look into it; pray over it; and follow your heart."

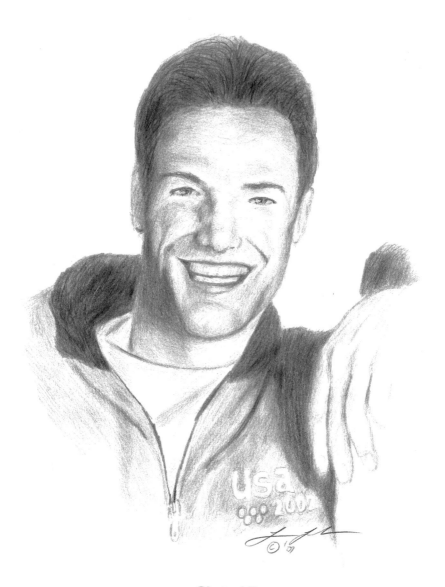

Chris Klug
Liver Recipient

5

Bronze-Medal Performance...
Gold-Medal Story
By Tim Mutrie

PARK CITY, Utah – Even though it ends happily ever after, Chris Klug's story reads more like an epic than a fairy tale.

We meet our hero following a disappointing sixth-place finish in snowboarding's 1998 Olympic debut at Nagano, Japan. He vows a return, a podium showing. At the time, he knows he's living with a degenerative liver disease, but he doesn't tell anyone except loved ones. No worries, he thinks. He was diagnosed years earlier, in 1993, during a routine physical. The endgame is transplant, doctors tell him, but that could be 20 or 30 years away. I'm healthy, I feel perfect, I'll be OK, he thinks. A blown-out knee later that winter, which knocks him out for the following season, weighs more heavily on his mind.

Klug comes back (the recurring theme of our saga). On Jan. 14, 2000, at Berchtesgaden, Germany, he rides to his second World Cup victory in alpine snowboarding. (It's the hard-boot racing the Euros dominate, not the tricky freestyle version, where Americans rule.) Four months later, he's surfing with friends and teammates in California, winding down from the season, when he's stricken with stabbing pains in his side. It's the liver. It's not working anymore. Doctors upgrade him to No. 1 on the transplant wait list. Three more months pass and our hero is slowly dying, but everyone holds out hope.

Then, in July 2000, a 13-year-old Westminster, Colo., boy dies, accidentally shot in the eye by a 14-year-old neighbor. The boy's parents make the decision to donate their son's organs. We hear all this later, of course, but Klug gets a new liver. His recovery is stunning, not a single rejection bout, and he's back on the snow three months later. He notes, however, that for the first time in his life, snowboarding isn't the most important thing anymore. Family and friends are, and he says he's stronger for it.

Six months later, almost exactly a year after the Berchtesgaden victory, Klug climbs back atop a World Cup podium at Kronplatz, Italy. It's a miracle, he says, and he believes it. And while he must take anti-rejection medication for the rest of his life, the prognosis is still good.

The 2002 Olympic season holds further challenges — on the snow, thankfully. Klug is off his mark in the early going, during the critical Olympic-team-qualifying events. His Olympic return begins to look doubtful. But true to form over the past two seasons, Klug is on in January, clinching the Olympic starting slot in the last two-out-of-five qualifiers. Not the way I would've written it, he says, but another character-building experience, just the same.

Nobody picks Klug as an Olympic favorite, but his face abounds in the media anyway because his story is so compelling. That's OK, Klug says, I want to get the message out about organ-donor issues. If I can use my celebrity to further that cause, I'm happy to do it, he says. In the week leading up to the Olympics, Klug grants one set of interviews that require a 2 a.m. wake-up call in order to appear on the East Coast morning shows. Today Show host Katie Couric later mentions his pin – an official Olympic "National Donor Day" pin, complete with the image of a snowboarder carving a turn – as one of the hottest pins at the Winter Games.

He exudes a quiet confidence before the parallel giant slalom event opens for qualifying on Thursday, Feb. 14 – coincidentally, National Organ Donor Awareness Day. Klug says he's riding as well as he ever has, he knows the hill at Park City as well as any slope in the world, and that the training the U. S. Team had on the hill in the previous weeks (before any other competitors arrived) is going to give him a huge advantage.

He then dedicates his Olympic performance to the donor family – "I wouldn't be here if it wasn't for their decision," he says – and to his sick grandmother, Ann McMahon, who couldn't make the trip. "And I'm representing Aspen and all the people who supported me and helped me get here," he adds.

Shifting Gears

More than 50 of Klug's friends and family made the seven-hour trek from Aspen to Salt Lake City for the two-day competition. Jim Klug, Chris' older brother, brought several dozen oversized blue-foam No. 1 fingers, stamped with "Team U. S. A. Chris Klug" in white, as well as "Chris Klug 2002 Winter Olympics" pins, with Klug's photo in the center. Coupled with the "Klug Riding" stickers plastered on Klug clan coats, and American flag tattoos decorating pensive cheeks, their presence in the finish area was unmistakable.

In Thursday's qualifying round, the field of 32 riders is cut in half, leaving the 16 fastest qualifiers to battle in the head-to-head, single-elimination finals on Friday, Feb. 15.

Starting from the unenviable No. 1 position Thursday morning, Klug posted the 11th fastest time, 37.17 seconds, 1.48 back from the leader, Gilles Jaquet of Switzerland (35.69). Austria's Alexander Maier, brother of World Cup champion alpine skier Hermann, was second (36.28), followed by Sweden's Daniel Biveson (36.42). But in parallel giant slalom, known as PGS, the winner is the racer who never loses, not necessarily the fastest rider on the hill.

"We got the job done. I'm in, and the game goes on," Klug said after racing Thursday. "And now the real fun starts."

"I'm one step closer to my goal now, and I've got another gear if I need it. I couldn't be in a better position."

In the finals, racers are paired off according to their qualifying times: No. 1 faces No. 16, No. 2 faces No. 15, and so on. The pairs then race simultaneously against each other in two runs, switching courses after the first run, with the faster rider advancing to the next round based on the total two-run time. Eventually, only two men remain to decide who rides off with the gold and who settles for silver.

Final Chapter

The Comeback Kid's roller-coaster ride of a race to

the bronze medal mirrored the drama of his life away from snowboarding.

"It's a miracle and a dream come true," Klug said following his final race. "What else can you ask for? A year-and-a-half ago, we're lying on our backs thinking we weren't going to live, and here we are now with a bronze medal around our necks. I still can't believe it."

But Klug's family and friends weren't as shocked. The contingent of family, friends and even doctors, staked out in the finish area all day waving the blue foam fingers in a frenzy each time he came down, were excited, yes, but not surprised.

"He's always had to overcome challenges since he was born, health wise, so we're not surprised at all," said brother Jim. "Whatever it takes, he's going to do it. That's the story of his life."

Aside from the Klug clan, few predicted Klug would even make it to the finals as he clearly struggled this season. His best World Cup PGS result was eighth place, and he only qualified for the Olympics at the last minute.

"All the magazines in the last couple weeks have come out and said he's a long shot for a medal," said Klug's mom Kathy, a teacher at Aspen High School. "I read it all and I'll tell you the truth, I said to myself, 'They don't know my son.'"

"Coming in nobody picked me for the podium," added Klug, "and that was fine with me. Like I've said before, I've gone up against worse odds. But after I qualified, I didn't care where I was (seeded) because I knew I had another gear and I was able to continue to play the game."

On the road to the bronze, Klug narrowly beat Canada's Jerome Sylvestre by .05 seconds to advance to the quarter-final round.

In Klug's second heat of that quarter-final round, against Walter Feichter of Italy, he took a wide line on the top steep section and fell behind. Then while trying to make up time on the flats at the bottom, Klug washed out on a heel side turn and lost by a hefty .75 seconds. But in the second run, Feichter missed a gate in the transition out of the steeps, affording Klug a comfortable cruise into the final four.

"A lot of the adversity I've faced in the last few years, I knew it'd work out in the end," Klug said, "and I've been reminded of it in the last few weeks. Before I got the transplant, I was getting sicker and sicker and I was starting to think I might not make it. But I kept the attitude that the window was still open; I'm not dead yet. And that was true yesterday when I was down to Feichter – the window's still open and I'm not giving up. That's what the Olympics are all about."

Klug's run at the gold medal halted in the semifinal round. Facing Swiss rider Philipp Schoch – the eventual gold medalist – Klug got loose on the steeps and entered the flats trailing by half-a-gate length. Klug never found his rhythm, washing out around several gates, and lost by 1.49 seconds, an eternity in PGS. In the deciding second run against Schoch, on opposite courses this time, Klug charged out of the start hut, aggressively trying to reel him in and advance to the gold-medal final. The tactic sent Klug into the fence and out of contention for the gold.

"He was riding pretty strong, and I had to have two good runs," Klug said of Schoch. "Then I started with a deficit in the second run, and I took some chances and ended up in the fence."

Schoch advanced to the gold-medal finals against Richard Richardsson of Sweden, while Klug dropped into the bronze-medal final versus France's Nicolas

Huet.

"It wasn't easy putting it (the semifinal loss) behind me, but I had to," Klug said. "I'd worked too hard to come up with no medal and come up short. I was obviously frustrated, but I had to move on. I didn't want to come home with fourth place – my goal's been to get on the podium after what happened in Nagano."

In the first run against Huet, Klug was cleaner and faster than his two bobbled runs against Schoch. Still, Huet enjoyed a slight lead in the first run until Klug shifted gears at the very bottom and sped ahead to win by .15 seconds.

During the run, Klug broke an instep buckle on his rear boot. Klug and ski tech Jay Cooper tried to replace it, but couldn't.

"We couldn't get the buckle off and the start referee is counting down, like 70 seconds and before I knew it he said 30 seconds and we didn't have the damn thing fixed. Finally, we put a pipe fastener on it with some duct tape; a total jerry-rig. But that's how I started, with my moon boots and duct tape 19 years ago, so it's only fitting that in the bronze-medal finals I had to rely on duct tape again," Klug chuckled.

After nearly forgetting his gloves, Klug said he put the buckle problem out of his mind. "I said to hell with it. I'm riding too good to have this one buckle derail me from a medal."

The fix held for the final run to determine the bronze medalist – Klug and Huet's eighth racing run of the day – and Klug ran away with a 1.36 second, combined victory.

As the only American in the field, fans in the base area rallied around him all day. And when Klug clinched the hardware, the place erupted.

"They were really supportive and it made a huge difference for me."

"This could be my biggest comeback yet, yeah, it may just be," Klug acknowledged. "But I may have another one in me. We'll see. I'd like to come back in four years and upgrade my medal."

On Friday night, Klug wore his medal to bed, all 15 minutes worth, as a party for Klug at the U. S. A. House in Park City ran all night.

"Everyone's lost their voices," he said. "It's hysterical. It's all sign language around here."

"The way today's events went are a good example of Chris," noted Aspen Club trainer Bill Fabrocini, who helped Klug rehab from knee surgery, then the transplant operation. "And the bronze medal is more meaningful than the gold because he had to fight for it."

"He was up and down, and he had to keep fighting," continued Fabrocini, who was in the crowd Friday. "It's the same thing with his knee rehab. At the time, we didn't know how far back he could come. And before the liver transplant, we didn't know what to expect either. But he kept fighting and believing, and when he didn't believe enough, [longtime girlfriend] Missy April believed for him, and his friends believed for him, and it's just like today when he was down. We all knew he was going to do it."

By Tim Mutrie
(First published in Aspen Times, Feb. 22, 2002)
Reprinted by permission

Liver

The liver is one of the largest and most complex organs in the body. It weighs about one pound in adults and is made up of a spongy mass of wedge-shaped lobes. The liver has numerous functions that are necessary for life. The liver 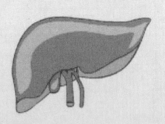 helps process carbohydrates, fats and proteins, and stores vitamins. It processes nutrients absorbed from food in the intestines and turns them into materials that the body needs for life. For example, it makes the factors that the blood needs for clotting. It also secretes bile to help digest fats, and breaks down toxic substances in the blood such as drugs and alcohol. The liver is also responsible for the metabolism of most drugs.

© United Network of Organ Sharing. Reprinted by permission.

U.S. Liver Transplants Performed

The chart below shows the number of liver transplants performed each year from 1997 to 2006.

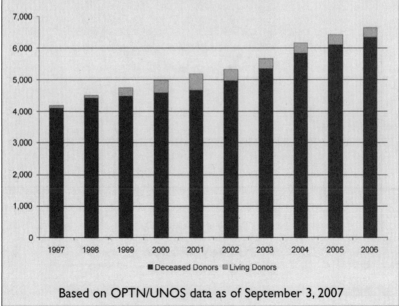

Based on OPTN/UNOS data as of September 3, 2007

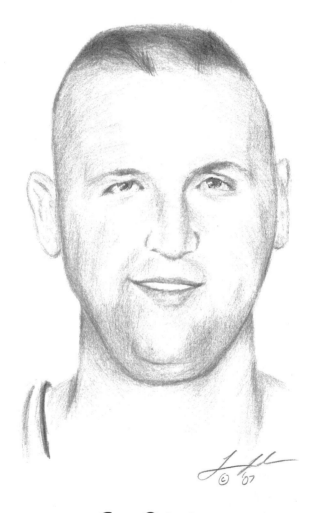

Greg Ostertag
Kidney Donor

A Gigantic Assist

By Joe Davidson

Amy Hall wants to get one thing perfectly clear, right out of the gate.

Just because she received her brother's 13-centimeter gift in a transplant doesn't mean her blood rages to the same temperature. Or that over the past two years the kidney injected any more country, any more twang to the slang.

Hall's only sibling is Greg Ostertag, the Kings' backup center and a 7-foot-2, 280-pound mass of Wrangler jeans and belt buckles, huntin' stories and guffaws. Brother and sister look a little alike, sound a lot alike and share the same fervent passion from crude jokes to Dolly Parton to family.

But that's it. She'll tell you that she's 6 feet of designer skirts, nice fashion, mean curves and good taste.

"Look, we're really close, but remind the people in Sacramento that I'm much better looking, I don't have his big (butt), and I'm a lot smarter," Hall said by phone from her office in Dallas, where she works in the accounting department for a law firm. "And I love my Ford dual-cab truck just as much as Greg loves his, only mine isn't a diesel, and I don't have a gun rack or mudflaps."

Theirs was always an unbreakable bond, 'Tag and kid sister.' He would hoist her high in the back yard of their Duncanville, Texas, home so she could peek at the puppies next door. They'd bicker and banter, fuss and fight, hug and howl.

The connection was made stronger and more lasting when Ostertag donated a kidney, since hers were failing from her struggle with diabetes.

Hall recovered fully, and Ostertag has shown no ill effects despite the rigors of NBA play. Hall counts every day as "a blessing" but understand this about this pair: No amount of surgery was going to sever their funny bone.

And when they talk on the phone today, it won't be a conversation with sappy Thanksgiving thoughts amid tears and reflection. Ostertag always begins conversations with his sister with, "How's Junior?" Junior, of course, is the kidney.

Before Junior, Hall didn't know if she'd have a future.

She was in dire straits in 2002 at age 29. She woke up one day blind in her right eye. She could barely muster the strength to get across the kitchen floor. She was, in effect, dying. She needed a kidney transplant, one of two bean-shaped organs the size of a fist that help rid the body of wastes. Ostertag was a perfect match, a rarity for some siblings, and he never hesitated to donate one of his two.

"Every day I'm thankful, so Thanksgiving isn't more prominent than any other day," Hall said. "Every day I get out of bed is an extra day I might not have had. Greg may say it's not a big deal because he's like that, but deep down, we both know it's a huge deal.

"It hasn't always been easy. I can't have kids. That's the path God has chosen for me. I've accepted it. But I'm very lucky and happy because I choose to be that way. Attitude is everything. I'm blessed to be here, and Greg is the reason."

Ostertag downplays his role. He's the only NBA player who gave a kidney in the middle of his career. Doctors have told him he needs no protective gear but must stay hydrated.

"She needed one, I had an extra, so I thought, what the heck?" Ostertag said. "She's a great gal, doing fine. The only way I'm really at risk is if I fall out of a tree huntin' or get hit by a truck."

Or if his sister lets him have it.

Hall said she will give her brother the business, reminding that she spent a good portion of her Tuesday night yelling at her TV, "Get your big butt in the paint, Greg!" That was Ostertag's best outing yet with the Kings – 14 minutes, five points, two rebounds against the Houston Rockets – since he signed with the team as a free agent last summer.

He'll roll with the critique.

About the only time these two get serious or somber is when they really talk about how dire things were for Hall.

She's more open to the topic than is her brother. Transplants and patient plights have become her life.

She regularly volunteers for speaking engagements on the importance of being a donor. She serves as a mentor for people who need a transplant and are on waiting lists in Dallas, offering encouragement and proof that things can get better, that a strong will and attitude are everything.

Ostertag isn't a kidney activist verbally, but he does have a T-shirt draped over his locker-room stall that tells of his loyalty. It reads, "An organ donor (me) saved my sister's life."

Hall recalled trying to muster the strength to make that call in February 2002. It's not every day someone asks her basketball brother for an organ that could end his career.

"I felt incredible guilt," Hall said. "You don't want to ever have to ask a sibling for something like this. What if one of his three kids needed one down the road, and he couldn't help them? Could I really do this to him?"

Hall knew it had to be some sort of good omen. Generally when she tries to call her brother at home, he doesn't answer because he's out on the land. This time, he answered. He calmed her.

"She was hysterical," Ostertag recalled.

Ostertag never gave a second thought to the prospect of walking away from some $16 million of salary from the Utah Jazz or someday facing the grim prospect of being unable to spare a kidney if one of his children needed a donor.

He told his Utah coaches and team management, "Look, my sister's in real trouble. I've got to help her."

When the 2001-02 season concluded, when all six tissue markers were a match, plans for the surgery in June were set in motion.

The basic rule of genetics among siblings, Hall recalled, is that "there was only a 25 percent chance that we'd match, but we did."

Ostertag knows why they matched: "We're twins,

only I'm two years older."

And the nurses needed a mop to absorb all the tears at the news this might work.

"Amy cried like a baby, so did my mom, and so did my dad," Ostertag said. "I didn't. OK. I lied. I cried, too. I couldn't help it."

Hall was told she might feel better within two weeks of the transplant. The prospect of feeling better at all – let alone in two short weeks – seemed dim. But within 10 days, she had noticed a difference.

"I felt like a million bucks, completely different," Hall said.

She still requires four insulin shots a day just as she has since she was 7 – "like brushing teeth, you're so used to it," she said. She has to take 57 pills a day to ward off side effects, infection, rejection.

Hall competed in a transplant Olympics basketball tournament in Minneapolis over the summer. She muscled inside, scored and rebounded. She also pleaded the importance of being a donor at clinics.

"If I get one person to take a donor card with them, then I've done my deed," she said.

What pains her, however, is greeting the sad people struggling to get through each day at the Baylor Medical Center in Dallas, where she had her transplant and where she mentors others.

"I talked to a guy who has been waiting 15 years for a kidney," she said." He's got a brother who is a match, but the brother won't do it because he's afraid. It breaks my heart."

Nationwide, 41 percent of living donor kidneys come from siblings, so Hall knows how important it can be for family members to be willing.

Said Ostertag: "There's no reason to be scared. I'm proof of that."

Ostertag's teammate, Peja Stojakovic, has a brother, Nenad, who has undergone two kidney transplants. The All-Star reports that his brother is doing fine, thanks to someone who was willing to donate.

"We feel lucky because none of us in the family were a match, and we all tried," Stojakovic said. "I admire Greg for what he's done. He gave his sister life."

The transplant also gave Ostertag a new image. For years, he was labeled everything from potential All-Star to underachiever to chief resident in coach Jerry Sloan's doghouse in Utah.

"I've been heckled my whole life," Ostertag said.

But after the transplant, things changed. No one challenged his heart anymore. Fans who jeered him in other NBA cities suddenly cooled it. They thrust a hand out or congratulated him verbally for being so heroic.

He was moved.

When a television commentator said he was tired of the story last year, that any sibling would have donated a kidney, Hall was incensed. She called the station in Minnesota, tracked down the commentator and told him stories of those in need under her mentorship. He apologized.

When Ostertag ran into that commentator later, he asked with a smile, "So, how's your (butt) feel after Amy chewed on it for a while?"

Shortly after Hall's transplant Olympics tour, she learned that the sore, swollen toe on her left foot was indeed broken. She had kicked a curb after climbing out of a car, feeling like a ballet dancer trying to dance with cowboy boots on.

Within days, she learned her brother had broken his hand, during the Kings' training camp, by falling at home.

She called, they swapped stories. They laughed. And

yes, Junior was fine.

"I guess both of us breaking a bone like that had something to do with the kidney, had to be," Hall said. "It's being a klutz from both ends of the spectrum, forever linked."

By Joe Davidson
(First published in the Sacramento Bee. Nov. 25, 2004)
Reprinted by Permission

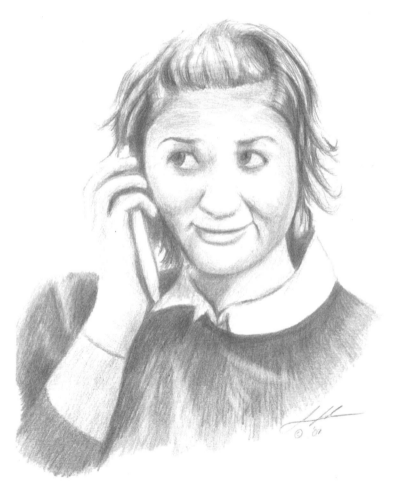

Allyson Thadeus-Zappe
Double Lung Recipient

7

Allyson Gets A Great Deal

What could be better than winning $124,000 on a television game show? For Allyson Thadeus-Zappe, the answer is easy. Although Allyson is thrilled to have won a six-figure prize on NBC's hit show "Deal or No Deal," she is even happier because of what had happened a few months before she appeared on the program. Allyson was happy to be alive.

Four months before her television debut, Allyson was on the waiting list for a lung transplant. She knew her condition was critical, and that she didn't have much time left. She told her husband, "If I don't get lungs while I am in the hospital now, I'm going to die."

At 16 months old, Allyson was diagnosed with cystic fibrosis, a genetic disease that causes mucus to build up in the lungs. The disease can result in life-threatening infections and serious digestive problems.

During her youth, Allyson was able to manage the

disease, even as a cheerleader for the Westlake (Ohio) High School Demons. As she matured, though, her disease worsened. At age 19, she was admitted to the hospital for the first of what would become a long string of hospitalizations.

"Ever since that first time, I was in the hospital at least once a year," Allyson said.

And the greatest moment of her life – giving birth to her daughter, Olivia – caused her disease to intensify dramatically. Allyson acknowledges that "the pregnancy and childbirth robbed me of everything." She knew her options were extremely limited: either a lung transplant or death.

The disease progressed to the point where Allyson could walk only one or two steps without stopping to sit down and rest, gasping for breath. "It was awful," she said, "I was sleeping 18 hours a day."

Unable to do much for herself, Allyson had to rely on her husband, Jim, who had to become both Mom and Dad to Olivia.

Allyson was fortunate to live long enough for a pair of lungs to become available. After a 10-month wait, she received a double lung transplant at the Cleveland Clinic in January 2006. The recovery was quick: She was discharged and went home after only 10 days.

"Brand new, beautiful lungs," Allyson said. "There is no way to describe how I felt."

Only four weeks after her transplant, Allyson learned about auditions for the television game show, "Deal or No Deal." She knew that her story might help her land a spot on the show. Although still present, the pain from the transplant was bearable, and Allyson was determined to try out.

The call telling her she had been selected as a contestant came on April 1. Initially, Allyson was sure it was an April Fool's prank.

On the day of the show, Allyson, like the other contestants, was told to bump fists rather than shaking hands with the show's notoriously germophobic host, Howie Mandel. Allyson says that approach "was just fine with me because I had just had my transplant and I had to be a germophobe at that point, too." During the show, Allyson's smile and vibrant personality won the hearts of the entire audience. She so dominated the show that even Howie seemed like a bit player.

The game format requires a banker to phone Howie with an offer of money to have the contestant quit the game, but Allyson would have none of that. At one point, she took control of the game, taking the phone call directly from the banker.

Howie had no choice but to stand by in amazement. Even while being upstaged, the germophobic host was so enamored with Allyson's energy that, at one point, he spontaneously gave her a hug.

Throughout the game, Allyson consulted her family for advice on whether to take the deal or risk it for a better offer. Her mother, Liz, said, "It's easy for me to tell her not to take (the deal). I'm already rich because I've got my baby back. No amount of money could compete with that."

Although Allyson started out slowly on the show, missing the $1 million prize with her second pick, she continued to get better offers. She eventually settled for the $124,000 although, had she stayed in the game until the end, she would have won $300,000.

Still, she says, "I'm very happy with the results."

Before the transplant, Allyson wouldn't have dreamed of being able to participate in a television game show. She simply would not have had the energy. With the transplant, however, Allyson is putting her newly acquired energy to the test, participating in an endless parade of meaningful activities.

"I've started a new job, I'm president of the PTA, I'm on the CF fundraising committee, I can play with Olivia and do things I could never do before," she boasts. Not bad for someone who a few months ago had to sleep 18 to 20 hours a day.

Now, Allyson keeps her life in perspective and speaks about her game show experience. "Had I won only a penny, had I won a million, the experience would have been awesome. Because I have a transplant, I have a whole new lease on life," Allyson said.

Always appreciative of the lungs she received, Allyson hopes her story will inspire others to become organ donors. She encourages others to speak with their families and make known their desires to be a donor.

Allyson hopes to be a donor when she dies and, as a mother, "would be more than honored, if something happened to Olivia, to donate her organs, because she could save as many as eight people. Let your family know your wishes. Let them know you want to be an organ donor."

Lung

The lungs are a pair of highly elastic and spongy organs in the chest. They are the main organs involved in breathing. They take in air from the atmosphere and provide a place for oxygen to enter the blood and for carbon dioxide to leave the blood. The lungs are divided into sections, with three on the right and two on the left.

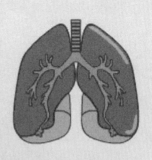

© United Network of Organ Sharing. Reprinted by permission.

U.S. Lung Transplants Performed

The chart below shows the number of lung transplants performed each year from 1997 to 2006.

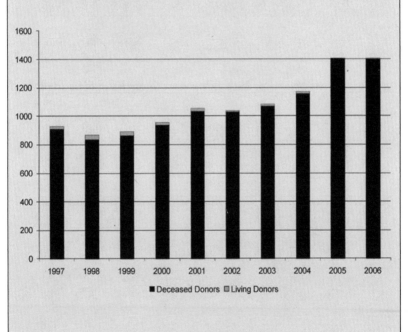

Based on OPTN/UNOS data as of September 3, 2007

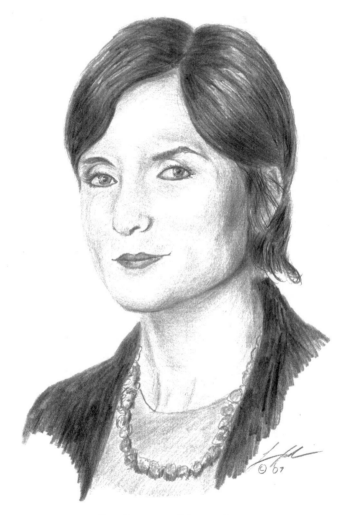

Catherine Herridge
Liver Donor

8

Fox News Correspondent's Living Donor Transplant Saved Her Infant Son
By Monica Haynes

Fox News correspondent Catherine Herridge is fearless.

Not because she's covered wars in Iraq and Yugoslavia.

No, her courage comes courtesy of a rosy-cheeked little miracle named Peter.

Five months ago, Peter, Herridge's infant son, was in desperate need of a liver. The family came to Children's Hospital of Pittsburgh. When tests determined that his mother was a good match, she donated a portion of her liver to her baby.

Now back on the air, Herridge, Fox's homeland defense correspondent, is sharing her story as a way of giving hope to other families facing a similar medical crisis.

"I had no idea until I was in this situation that there was such a shortage of organs, especially for small children," said Herridge, 42. "I look at Peter, and he is pink and he has big fat cheeks and he has five teeth coming in, and I cannot believe that my liver is inside him and that's why it's happening."

Peter was born in December with biliary artesia, a rare chronic liver disease in which the bile ducts are blocked, causing progressive damage to vital body functions.

In April, Peter, his parents and 2-year-old brother, Jamie, came to Pittsburgh, where the baby was placed on the transplant list. At one point, Herridge said, the family thought a liver might be available for Peter, but it went to a child who was even sicker than he.

In May, his mother was screened, and doctors determined she would be an ideal candidate for a living donor transplant. Still, they wanted to wait until the beginning of June to see if a donor liver would become available.

"In our case, the ideal situation is one where a parent can donate because genetically you're so close," Herridge said.

But there are other factors as well. The donor must have a matching blood type and he or she must be in good health and of compatible size. Despite the obvious difference between adult and baby, Herridge, who is 5 feet, 4 inches, is closer in size to Peter than her husband, JD, who is more than 6 feet tall.

On June 6, surgeons at UPMC Presbyterian, in a seven-hour procedure, cut a foot long incision and removed 20 percent of Herridge's liver. It was then taken down the street to Children's Hospital and implanted in Peter during a 10-hour surgery.

"I remember when I woke up, the first thing I asked

the doctor was, 'Did you get my liver, and did you give it to Peter?'" she recalled.

Dr. George V. Mazariegos, director of pediatric transplantation at Children's Hospital, led the surgical team that conducted Peter's transplant.

"Actually, the data suggests that a living donation may be even the best option, particularly for a very small child under age 1," he said. "Despite the fact that's technically challenging to do, those livers function very well."

Children's Hospital does about 50 pediatric liver transplants a year, Dr. Mazariegos said. Thirty of those involve only the liver; 20 include both liver and intestines.

Like all transplant patients, Peter must take an anti-rejection medicine, and for the first three months he needed monthly lab checks. Now, his Pittsburgh doctors won't need to see him for another three months, Dr. Mazariegos said. If everything checks out after that, he will undergo annual checkups.

"We're very excited that he has a prognosis for an excellent long-term recovery," Dr. Mazariegos said.

Herridge can see the evidence of that. "He is really a lot healthier today than he was three months ago," she said. "He's growing well. He was happy before; he's super happy now."

Peter, who spent a third of his life lying on his back in the hospital, has a little catching up to do to reach the developmental level of his fellow 9-month-olds. But he is trying to crawl now, she said, and by the time he's 18 months, he should be pretty much caught up.

During the ordeal, Fox's Greta Van Susteren aired her colleague's story and kept viewers updated via her blog.

"We do so many stories that are very distressing,

war, murder, missing people," Van Susteren said. "I'm immensely impressed by what modern medicine can do for catastrophic things."

She said she began to hear that Peter might have a medical problem after her co-worker didn't return as scheduled from maternity leave. The two newswomen talked, and Herridge told Van Susteren about the option of donating a portion of her liver to her son.

"When she finally found out she could do something, she was full speed ahead, no question about it," Van Susteren said.

The broadcast garnered a lot of response from families with children in the same situation, many of them unaware that a living donor transplant was possible, she said.

"I also continue to hear from families whose children have liver disease and are facing transplants," she said. "I've spoken to some of these families and corresponded with them."

While the operation was a success, Fox news editors had discussions about the possibility of a not-so-good outcome. "Some of it was done without me present, I found out later," Van Susteren said. "My view is that even if it hadn't turned out well, I was still inspired."

She said she was stunned by how hard the doctors and nurses at Children's worked and how dedicated and caring they are.

"When I was in the hospital with Peter, talking to the surgeon the day before, when no one was looking I saw the surgeon stroking Peter's head and how much he loved that child," Van Susteren said.

"I knew these doctors day in and day out are saving lives. I had such faith in them even if we'd have an unfortunate result I still knew the story would be important for others."

Herridge said her colleague deserves a lot of credit for doing the story and encouraging people to make donations to the UPMC transplant fund. She said the hospital uses the money to help families buy anti-rejection medicine.

She said that she continues to get e-mails from people who've had transplants and encourage her to hang in there during that tough first year.

"I really feel more fearless in a lot of ways now than I did before," Herridge said.

"You cannot confront the possibility that your child can die and that you have to put yourself at risk to save them without being changed. There are not many things that would faze or frighten me now."

By Monica Haynes
Copyright, *Pittsburgh Post Gazette,* all rights reserved.
(First published by Pittsburgh Post-Gazette Sep. 26, 2006)
Reprinted by permission

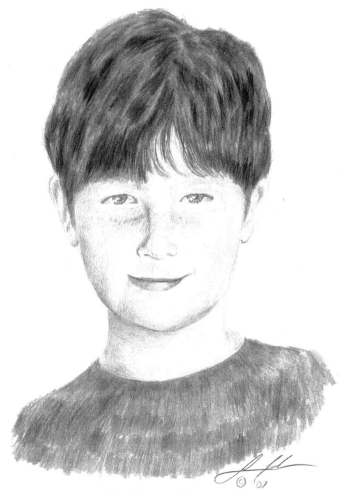

Nicholas Green
Organ and Cornea Donor

A Child's Legacy of Love
By Reg Green (Nichalas' Father)

Recently I strolled through a park in Rome with Andrea Mongiardo, a 23-year-old Italian, whose heart once belonged to my own son.

My son, Nicholas, a magical little creature, whose teacher said he was the most giving child she'd ever met, was 7 when he was shot thirteen years ago in a botched robbery on the main highway south from Naples. Two young men, mistaking our rental car for one they thought was carrying jewelry from Rome to stores in southern Italy, fired on us, hitting Nicholas in the head. Two days later he was declared brain dead.

I can remember that sunlit hospital room, with the doctors standing in a group in the corner, leaving my wife, Maggie, and me alone to absorb their terrible news and the thought that came with it: "How will I ever get through the rest of my life without him?"

Never to run my fingers through his hair again, never to tickle him or hear him say "Good night, Daddy."

We sat there numbly for a few more moments. Then one of us – we don't remember which but, knowing her, I'd guess Maggie – said, "Now that he's gone, shouldn't we donate the organs?" and the other said "yes." And that was all there was to it. Although we are not a gloomy family and still laugh a lot, every morning when I wake I know life will never have the sparkle it had when Nicholas was alive. But we have never had a moment's regret about our decision – and if we had had any regrets they would have been banished by the first sight of the seven recipients, four of them teenagers, whom we met a few months later.

None of the four teens could have expected to live much longer, two of the adults were going blind and the third, a diabetic, was in pitiful shape, her whole central nervous system disintegrating, scarcely able to see, unable to walk without help.

Andrea was all too typical. Born with a severely deformed heart, he stopped growing when he was 7. He underwent a dangerous operation, which failed, then another, which also failed, then a third, a fourth and a fifth. None of them worked. His family was in despair.

He became so sick he could scarcely walk to the elevator in his apartment building. Every other day he went to the hospital for a transfusion of albumin, the protein that kept him alive. He was hollow cheeked, a frightened look set on his face. At 15-years-old he knew he couldn't last much longer.

The turning point came in March 1994 when the doctors at Rome's Bambino Gesu (Baby Jesus) Hospital brought up the idea of a transplant. "Only a new heart can save him," they told his parents. At first he said no. After five failed operations he was understandably reluctant to have another.

But he was persuaded to try. He was put on the waiting list and began the long, cruel, double-edged wait that could only end successfully if someone else died. Seeing him now, and knowing what would have happened to him, I know that if we had made a different decision, and shrugged off his problems and those of the other recipients as none of our concern, neither Maggie nor I could ever have looked back without a deep sense of shame.

The operation was much more difficult than a normal transplant because of the acute deformation of his heart; he hung between life and death. At length, however, it was a resounding success. The new heart turned out to be a perfect match. "It might have been made for him," Lidia, his mother, told me, a tear in her eye since, being a mother, she never forgets the little boy it came from. Andrea has had his share of ups and downs, as his body, like that of all transplant recipients, tries to reject the new organ. But, all in all, he is thriving. He plays soccer, works with an uncle who manages condominiums and finds deep satisfaction in the simple things of life. Looking at him in a crowd you would never pick him out as the one who spent half his childhood in hospital. We would have done anything to keep Nicholas alive, of course. But that wasn't an option. So standing next to Andrea in the park, wasn't horrifying or depressing or awkward. We've never thought of Nicholas living on in any literal way inside him or the others but, as I put my arm round his shoulders, I did feel a kinship to Nicholas' pure heart, beating steadily, and a flow of satisfaction, knowing that even in death he continued to give so fully.

We first met our recipients and their families just a few months after the shooting, when our grief was still agonizingly raw. But that meeting, which both of us had to steel ourselves to attend, was explosive. A door opened and in came this mass of humanity, some smiling, some tearful, some ebullient, some bashful, a stunning demonstration of the momentous consequences every donation can have. We now think of them as an extended family. We've watched the children grow and leave school and get their driver's licenses and the adults go back to work. One of them, 19-year-old Maria Pia Pedala, in a coma with liver failure on the day Nicholas died, bounced back to good health, married and has since had a baby boy. And, yes, they have called him Nicholas.

In Italy schools, squares and the largest hospital have also been named for him. Better still, organ donation rates have almost tripled. Yet they still fall far below the need.

I have a story I like to tell about Nicholas. On our way to Italy a few days before he was killed, we played a game in which he was a Roman soldier returning home, after years heroically guarding the frontiers. When you get to Rome, we told him, you'll be famous. Poems will be written about you, streets will be named for you, you'll get a gold medal.

It was only a game. But it all came true. With this difference: that Nicholas conquered not by the force of arms but by the power of love and that, of course, is much stronger.

By Reg Green
(First published in the Los Angeles Times)
Reprinted by permission

Heart

The heart is a strong and muscular organ that is about the size of a fist in adults. It pumps blood throughout the body and is located behind the breastbone between the lungs. Deoxygenated blood flows from the heart to the lungs where it gives up carbon dioxide and is freshly oxygenated. From there, the blood returns to the heart and is pumped to the rest of the body.

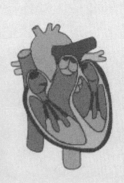

© United Network of Organ Sharing. Reprinted by permission.

U.S. Heart Transplants Performed

The chart below shows the number of heart transplants performed each year from 1997 to 2006.

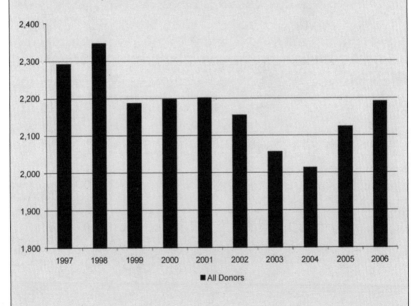

Based on OPTN/UNOS data as of September 3, 2007

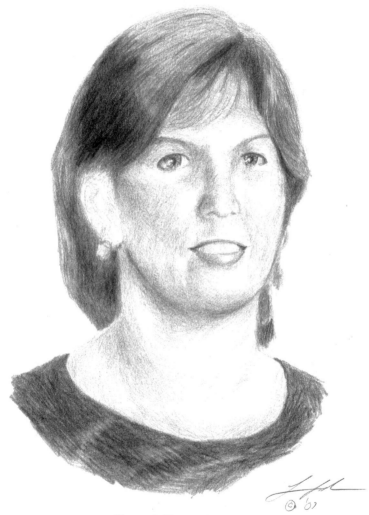

Peggi Rumsey
Lung Donor

10

Brian Gets His Second Wind

Peggi Rumsey found out almost by accident that a distant relative needed a lung transplant. While at another relative's house, Peggi found a form letter written by her former stepbrother, someone she had not seen in a very long time. The letter was a plea for someone to donate a lobe of a lung to his son, Brian. A cystic fibrosis sufferer, Brian was close to death and could be saved only with a lung transplant.

There was a small chance that a lung would become available from a deceased donor, but that chance was rare indeed. The waiting list was long, and Brian's time was short. In New York, where Brian lived, the average wait at the time was two years, and Brian had, at most, six months to live.

The procedure for transplanting lungs from a living donor is called a living donor lobectomy. It involves cutting a lobe of lung from each of two donors, with both lobes then transplanted into a single recipient. It is an extremely serious operation.

For the recipient, the surgery means the difference between life and death. The lungs diseased with cystic fibrosis must be completely removed so they do not infect the healthy, transplanted lungs. Then the two lung lobes are transplanted into the recipient's chest cavity.

Although the letter was not addressed to Peggi, she was moved to take action. She thought about Brian's plight for about 30 minutes, and then decided that, if she were healthy enough to donate, Brian could have a piece of her lung.

Although Peggi and Brian were related, they were certainly not close. She had not seen him for at least 10 years, the last time at a family reunion when their paths barely crossed. It had been such a long time ago, Peggi was not even sure if she would recognize Brian if they passed on the street.

Peggi's mother was once married to Brian's grandfather. Both parents had children from previous marriages, but had none together. And when the relationship ended, each family went its own way.

At first, there was some interaction between the children. They still saw each other on occasion, but they were not particularly close. After a few years of separation, fewer occasions brought them together. Eventually, they simply grew apart until they started their own families.

When Peggi's step-brother married and had two sons, Peggi would occasionally baby-sit the boys. Brian, the younger of the two, was diagnosed with cystic fibrosis as a baby.

This came as a shock to everyone, as neither parent knew they carried the recessive gene that caused the disease. Statistically, each child whose parents have this gene has a 25 percent chance of inheriting the disease. Brian's brother was healthy, but Brian was not so lucky.

A person afflicted with cystic fibrosis, which causes mucus to build up in the lungs, often requires treatments to dislodge the mucus by one of various methods. When Brian was a child, Peggi would occasionally help clear his lungs with a clap treatment, which required that Brian be turned upside-down and slapped vigorously on his back. The treatment would free the mucus from his lungs, allowing him to breathe once again.

Cystic fibrosis affects approximately 30,000 people in the United States. Those afflicted have a gene that causes them to produce abnormally thick mucus. The mucus clogs the lungs and is prone to supporting infections that are often life-threatening. In addition, the mucus prevents digestive enzymes required to breakdown food from reaching the intestines.

There is no cure for cystic fibrosis, but research is ongoing. There have been some positive results, but nothing to indicate that a cure is near. The best hope available is testing to determine whether the parents carry the recessive gene, allowing couples to know if there is a chance their children will be afflicted. This test was not available when Brian's parents got pregnant. His disease came as a total shock to everyone involved.

When he was young, Brian was active and kept his disease at bay. He was on the wrestling team at school and also kept busy with other athletic endeavors. Cystic fibrosis did little to slow him down until he reached his mid-teens, when it robbed him of his ability to remain active.

Most people with cystic fibrosis have shortened life

expectancies. The median survival age is 33.4 years, according to the Cystic Fibrosis National Data Registry. And, even here, Brian was being short-changed. At 20 years old, he was given only six months to live.

Cystic fibrosis is not usually carried on to the next generation. Ninety-five percent of the men with this disease are sterile. And, while some women with the disease can conceive, most cannot carry the baby to term. Limited lung function and other health factors prevent generations of people afflicted with this debilitating disease.

No one from Brian's biological family was considered suitable as a lung donor, and he could not survive the wait for a deceased donor. It looked as though Brian would not live. In a last desperate plea, Brian's father sent the form letter asking for a monumental gift – a lobe of a lung.

To qualify as a lung donor, the donor's blood type must be compatible with the recipient's. The donor must be in good physical shape, have normal pulmonary function and be three to six inches taller than the recipient for the lung to fit the chest cavity. A donor also must be willing to refrain from smoking for the rest of his or her life.

Four people, including Peggi, stepped forward and offered to be tested as potential donors. One was a wrestling teammate, Michael, who was also one of Brian's closest friends. Another was Michael's father, also a long-time friend. Preliminary testing quickly ruled out everyone but Michael and Peggi.

Before becoming donors, the two would have to undergo extensive testing. There are potentially severe risks to the donor, including infection, bleeding and pain. Some donors can experience prolonged leakage of either fluid or air. Despite the risks, both donors wanted to move forward. Even though Peggi did not know Brian well, she said, "If he died, I would not be able to live with myself. I had to do it."

Living lung donation is relatively rare. Few hospitals nationwide are equipped to perform this operation. For Peggy and Michael, the testing would take place at Brigham and Women's hospital in Boston.

Donor testing is quite extensive, requiring several trips to the hospital for evaluation. Although the distance between their homes in New York and the transplant center in Boston was not too far, it was far enough that it required Michael and Peggi to make overnight stays. Although this fact would cause a financial burden for Peggi and her family, what mattered was that Peggi had a chance to help save Brian's life. Everything else would have to take care of itself.

Peggi's husband, Edward, was completely supportive, standing behind his wife through the entire ordeal. He would have done the same thing if his wife were not able to do as she planned.

There were other challenges ahead, too. Peggi was a stay-at-home mom with two small children. She and Edward would have to find someone to care for the children while Peggi was on her mission to save Brian. But Peggi was determined to do what had to be done.

Peggi, who enjoyed exercising, belonged to a local gym. A good workout allowed her to burn off the tension of the day, and to relax and be herself. The gym had a daycare center that allowed her to drop off her four-year-old son, Jason, while she worked out. It was a good arrangement; Jason loved the play area. The workout sessions were a treat for both mother and son.

As Peggi's testing progressed, she became more open in her discussions about her life. She mentioned to her gym instructor, Adeline, that she was intent on donating part of her lung. Impressed that anyone would make such a sacrifice for a person she hardly knew, Adeline took a personal interest, offering to do "whatever she could" to help Peggi through the ordeal.

As the surgery drew near, Peggi became more and more concerned about her children. The couple did not have the financial resources to allow Edward to take time off work, and Peggi would not be strong enough after surgery to take care of Jason and his sister, Ellie. Although Ellie, at age seven, would be in school during the work day, someone would have to care for Jason while Peggi recovered and her husband continued to work.

Peggi turned to Adeline. When Adeline offered to do whatever she could, Peggi, haltingly asked, "Could you help with the kids?" Adeline agreed without hesitation. This was so little to ask for a person so giving.

Whenever Peggi needed to be away from home for testing, Adeline stepped in. When Adeline had to work, she took Jason with her and let him play in the daycare center, a real treat for him. And when she wasn't working, she came over to the house to cook and do whatever needed to be done. Peggi felt as though Mary Poppins had floated into her life.

As the process progressed, problems arose. It became apparent that the Boston transplant team was not ready to take on such a difficult surgery. They had done lung transplants before, but only once with living donors. A lung donation from living patients required three operating rooms running simultaneously.

Brian, meanwhile, was getting closer to death. His doctor looked for another transplant center with more experience in the procedure, one better equipped to perform the surgery. UCLA looked most promising at first, but the distance and Brian's poor health made it impossible to seriously consider the facility.

Eventually the group identified Duke University in North Carolina, which had experience with living lung donation and was willing to look at Brian's case. On February 16, his 21st birthday, Brian was rushed to Duke University Medical Center to determine whether he could survive the surgery.

Michael and Peggi remained in New York waiting for a call. If Brian were deemed healthy enough, the surgery would be scheduled for the following Friday. If he were not healthy enough, there was no back-up plan. Brian was simply running out of time.

Unable to know whether the surgery was going forward, Peggi couldn't book a flight in advance. If she received word the surgery would take place, she would have to get to North Carolina quickly, and it would be expensive. But the cost, although important, was the least of her worries. There was a life hanging in the balance, and she was willing to do whatever she could to keep Brian alive.

The Duke team evaluated Brian and determined he was strong enough for the transplant. After also reviewing Peggi's and Michael's test results, the team determined the surgery was worth the risk.

On the Internet, Peggi had found Angel Flight, an organization of private pilots that fly patients in need of medical attention. She told them of her situation, and they happily agreed to get her to North Carolina in time for the operation.

Peggi met the airplane at a small airport near her home. The pilot, Richard Schuster, owned a small turbojet. Angel Flight gave him an excuse to fly as he helped patients in need of medical attention. Richard would get Peggi to Baltimore, where another pilot would meet them and fly her to North Carolina.

The plans, however, were interrupted. The weather in Baltimore had turned sour and the pilot who met them there had a much smaller plane that was not as well equipped to handle the storm. The plane had only a single engine, and the pilot knew its limitations. He couldn't fly.

Having come this far, Richard refused to turn back. He would take Peggi the rest of the way. For Peggi, Angel Flight was the experience of a lifetime. She said, "I would definitely give up another organ to do this again."

Once everyone had arrived in North Carolina safely, a few more tests and evaluations were all that remained for the surgical team to ensure there were no changes that would threaten the surgery or decrease the chance of success. The lives of three people were on the line.

When the day of surgery arrived, the three patients were anxious. But, despite some fear and some worrisome moments, there was no hesitation. Both donors knew they had a rare opportunity to help save Brian's life. Brian knew this was his best, and perhaps only, chance to live.

Peggy and Michael, whose surgeries would start first, were taken to separate operating rooms while Brian waited in pre-op. He would be taken into surgery only after the surgeons were certain that the donor lung lobes could be safely removed without compromising the donors' health.

The lung lobes were taken without problem, and soon all three patients were undergoing delicate surgical procedures. A portion of Peggi's left lung was removed, as was a portion of Michael's right lung. Both of Brian's diseased lungs were removed.

Michael's and Peggi's healthy lung lobes were transplanted into Brian's chest and began functioning right away. The long road was nearing completion; the gamble had paid off. Brian would have a new lease on life.

Peggi had no side effects. Discharged from the hospital four days after surgery, she stayed in North Carolina for a few additional days to recover from her surgery – and figure out a way to get back home. She was not strong enough to fly, and her doctor would not allow it for fear that there would be a delay in getting her medical attention if a complication should occur. Though Angel Flight assured the physician they could have Peggi on the ground in 20 minutes if need be, the doctor felt her best means of transportation would be by car.

Peggi would have to wait a few more days until Brian's father could drive her back to New York. He was very anxious to help her get back home. His former stepsister had just saved his son's life. Although they had grown apart over the years, they now shared a very strong bond not likely to be broken.

The drive seemed longer to Peggi than the nine-and a half-hours it was. The pain made her quite uncomfortable, but she was happy to be going back home to recover with her family.

Within eight days of surgery, Peggi was back to cleaning house and working out at the gym. At first, things were slow as she rebuilt her strength, but it was not long before she was back to normal.

"It all seems so surreal to me. I only have photos to prove it really happened," Peggi said.

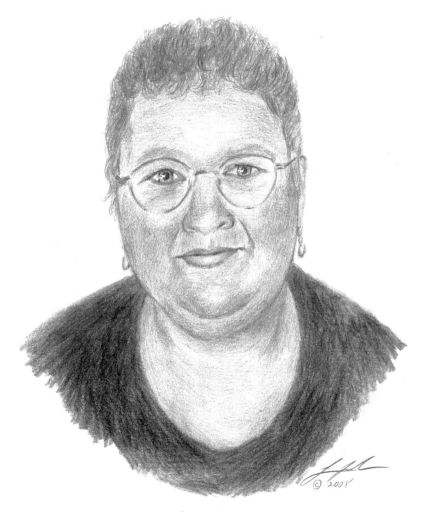

Sue Rebello
Pancreas Auto Islet Recipient

11

Relief at last

Although Sue Rebello suffered from chronic pain, she had trouble getting the help she needed. Her frequent visits to the emergency room did not resolve her problems. Sometimes she was given medication and sent on her way. Another time she was simply given a placebo – a sugar pill, hoping this would resolve the pain as if it was all in her head. The sugar pill convinced her that the emergency room was not the answer. So she suffered quietly while trying to endure the pain.

Doctors could not find the source of her pain. A biopsy of her liver showed nothing. Her gall bladder appeared to be normal, but yet the pain persisted. The doctors decided to remove her gall bladder hoping that would help. During surgery they learned her gall bladder was indeed diseased and inflamed, it had even become imbedded in her liver. Although the gall bladder was removed, the pain persisted. Sue still experienced chronic pain and no one knew the reason why.

Sue traveled to Boston hoping the doctors there would find the source of her problem. In Boston, it was determined that her pain was caused by pancreatitis. It was discovered that the accessory duct in her pancreas was missing – apparently she had been born without it. The pancreas is designed to release enzymes and help in the digestion of food. In Sue's case the pancreas created the enzymes, but they could not travel into the digestive system. The enzymes remained at the source, and began to digest the pancreas, causing her severe pain.

Doctors surgically inserted a stent in an attempt to release the enzymes from the pancreas. Even then, the stent became obstructed and within three weeks of surgery she was unable to stand due to intense pain. The stent had to be removed.

Over the next year, she was hospitalized three more times with the same unresolved problem. She spent more than twenty days in the hospital that year. On one occasion, she was given two units of blood. Still no relief.

Surgeons performed a surgical procedure dubbed the 'Whipple Procedure' in which the head of her pancreas was removed and a duct was created for the enzymes to pass. The tail of her pancreas was left in place allowing it to function normally.

The Whipple Procedure gave her some relief and she was able to go back to eating a small amount of food. Her good fortune did not last long, however. Right before Christmas, she checked back into the hospital for yet another holiday.

Over the next year, Sue tried another tack to control her pain – medication. It helped some, but still did not solve the problem. She loved her job and continued to work – when she could. She was determined to keep her job despite her frequent bouts with sickness, hospital-izations and pain. But in June 1997, it all came to an end. She was once again hospitalized and she had to leave her job.

Her next bout of pain occurred at the end of August, when she returned to the hospital once again. This time the pain was accompanied by anemia and malnutrition. She was hospitalized for twenty-one days. She said, "Every time they tried to introduce food, the beast inside me kicked up its heels into a frenzied attack." Everything she ate would cause her severe pain – even something as small as a half of a Popsicle.

It became obvious that her pancreas was not going to get any better. Doctors advised her to have her pan-creas removed entirely even though that would mean she would acquire diabetes. The pancreas produces insulin to help regulate blood sugar. Without a pan-creas, she would have to inject the insulin as many dia-betic people do. The chronic pain would be replaced with a dreaded disease. Her choices were thought to be limited.

Her primary care physician agreed with the doctors in Boston who had come to know her so well. She had already lost sixty pounds and was not getting the nour-ishment she needed. They gave her total parenteral nutrition (TPN) in which her only source of nourish-ment was liquid 'food' given to her through a feeding tube. Although Dr. McIlvaine, her primary care physi-cian agreed with the other doctors, she also informed her about an experimental and unproven procedure called a pancreatectomy with auto islet transplant.

Sue contacted Dr. David Sutherland at the University of Minnesota Medical Center, the pioneer of this procedure. With the procedure, Dr. Sutherland would remove the pancreas altogether, but would separate the islet cells from the pancreas and then return the islet cells to Sue's body. The theory was that the islet cells would produce the required insulin without the pain she had become accustomed to.

Accepting that she should have the pancreatectomy, Sue decided to take the chance with the auto islet transplant. After all, her pancreas would be gone in either case. If the islets produced insulin, she might be able to avoid diabetes. And if they didn't? She would be in the same condition as if she opted for the pancrectomy alone.

Before she could schedule the trip to Minnesota for the procedure, Sue returned to the hospital with another bout of pain. She was on TPN as her sole source of nutrition and required that a feeding tube be inserted until the surgery could be scheduled in Minnesota. Sue named her TPN apparatus 'Penelope' and it became her constant companion. She could go nowhere without it. By now Sue was down to 115 pounds and when full Penelope weighed eight pounds and was cumbersome to deal with. Penelope had to be strapped to a luggage cart to help Sue get through the airport on her way to Minnesota.

Sue was single and had to make the trip to Minneapolis alone. Her mother could not accompany her – she had just had surgery herself. A sorry sight, she befriended Mary, one of her flight attendants who took her under her wing. Sue considered Mary 'an angel sent to watch over her.' Mary even spent a few hours with her on Thanksgiving Day while she was so far from home.

The surgery took place in November and had an immediate affect. Within five days of the surgery, Sue was insulin free and not diabetic. Further, as the pain from surgery subsided, she learned the pain from pancreatitis was gone as well. Two weeks after surgery Sue's long ordeal was over. "Miracles do happen," she proclaimed.

After her surgery, it took time for Sue to gain back her strength. She takes enzymes by mouth after she eats or drinks to help her body digest food properly.

Sue has met other people who have had their pancreas removed, including one from Israel. "It's amazing how many people are struggling with this disease," she says. Sue is excited when she learns of another person who was suffering from chronic pancreatitis who decided "to bury the beast in them in the river in Minneapolis" – as she likes to call it.

"Looking back on things," Sue says, "I would have the pancreatectomy and auto islet transplant again in a heartbeat if I needed it. The only thing I would do differently is that I would have had it done sooner and, perhaps, not have had the Whipple procedure."

Ten Years Later:

Sue celebrated her 10th anniversary on November 17th, 2007. Ten years given back to a once frail body. Ten years of being able to eat whatever she likes without severe pain. Sue went a full 5 years with no signs of diabetes. After 5 years, Sue did become a diabetic but her diabetes is mild because she still has her islet cells transplanted into her liver. Without the transplant Sue would have been an uncontrollable diabetic. Diabetes runs in Sue's family and she feels she would have become diabetic even without her ordeal with pancreatitis.

Sue decided to retire early due to her many years of illness. She is living as normal a life as possible. Sue dedicates her time to communicating with other pancreatitis sufferers and educating them about the total pancreatectomy and auto islet transplantation. "It's just a wonderful feeling to know I have helped a fellow sufferer out," Sue exclaims.

Pancreas

The pancreas is a five to six inch gland located behind the stomach. The pancreas produces enzymes that are used for digestion, and insulin, which is essential for life because it regulates the use of blood sugar throughout the body.

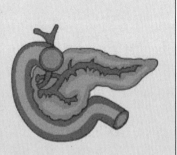

© United Network of Organ Sharing. Reprinted by permission.

U.S. Pancreas Transplants Performed

The chart below shows the number of pancreas transplants performed each year
from 1997 to 2006.

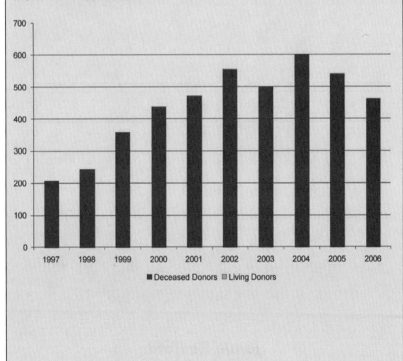

Based on OPTN/UNOS data as of September 3, 2007

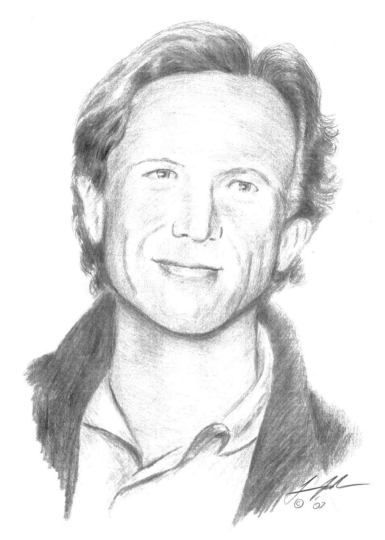

Jamie Redford
Liver Recipient

12

The Redford Family's Private Crisis

by Carrie St. Michel

"I remember waking up, and my entire family was standing in a semicircle around my hospital bed, holding hands. I will never forget it," says Jamie Redford. "In that instant, I realized the power of family – the power of family love."

It could have been one of those perfectly scripted movie moments that the patient's father plays so well. This, however, was no film set. On March 15, 1993, a painfully real drama was unfolding in the private lives of Hollywood legend Robert Redford and his family. The Redfords' son, Jamie, was fighting for his life, following sudden surgery to replace his liver.

At Jamie's bedside were his father, mother Lola Van Wagenen, sisters Shauna and Amy, and wife Kyle, engulfing him with love and support, just as they had through years of illness that began when he was 15.

Now, at 30, he had just returned from the brink of death.

Unfortunately, that first transplant was not the success doctors had hoped for; Jamie would have many more medical battles to fight. The long ordeal eventually led to a filmmaking effort of his own. Last year, the younger Redford completed *The Kindness of Strangers,* a gripping feature-length documentary exploring the miraculous, complex world of organ donation. It airs this month on HBO.

In a pleasant outdoor cafe near his Marin County, CA, home, Jamie, now 37, nervously readjusts his well-worn Sundance baseball cap as he recalls the struggle that spanned two decades of his life. It is a story few people know about, even though it began when his father was at the height of movie superstardom. The Redfords purposely shielded their children from the Hollywood spotlight, raising them in New York City and Sundance, UT.

Jamie was in the tenth grade when he first came down with what appeared to be a particularly acute case of stomach flu. There were grueling attacks of cramps, chills, fevers, and fatigue.

Throughout high school, Jamie would periodically feel well enough to hit the ski slopes, play guitar in a local rock band, and live like a normal teenager. Then the mysterious illness would reappear.

Robert and Lola Redford, who married in 1959, had already endured one terrible tragedy, losing their first child, Scott, to sudden infant death syndrome when he was just 3 months old. They resolved that they would not lose Jamie. They went from doctor to doctor, until finally, in 1980, their son's condition was diagnosed as ulcerative colitis – a chronic inflammatory disease of the large intestine that slowly destroys the colon.

Amid bouts of internal bleeding, rapid weight loss, and scorching fevers, Jamie managed to complete a bachelor's degree at the University of Colorado. Then, in 1987, he received a new, far more deadly diagnosis: primary sclerosing cholangitis (PSC) – a rare complication of ulcerative colitis that blocks the liver's bile ducts. "They told me my liver would fail within five to ten years," Jamie remembers.

Only 25 at the time, Jamie reacted with a healthy dose of denial. "I decided it wouldn't get me," he says. "They'd come up with a cure." His parents were less laissez-faire and immediately rushed to their son's aid. "They offered to fly me anywhere to get the right care and guided me to anything that could be of help," says Jamie. Though the Redfords had divorced two years earlier, in 1985, their son's illness overruled any tensions between the two. "You're always going to be parents to the same children," Lola has said. "Through all of this with Jamie, Bob and I really leaned on each other for a lot of emotional support."

Jamie, though, had something other than medical care on his mind. Two months after the PSC pronouncement, he proposed to Kyle Smith, whom he'd met at college. Without hesitation, she said yes, a fact that still amazes Jamie. "It never occurred to her what she was getting into," he observes. "Our lives were just one – what was happening to me was happening to her."

By 1989, Jamie was experiencing excruciating abdominal pains, "curled-up-on-the-ground kind of pains," as he puts it. In 1991, doctors said a "transplant would be needed sooner rather than later." By now the stakes had grown even higher. Jamie had become a father: Son Dylan was born that same year. (Now Jamie and Kyle also have a 3-year-old daughter, Lena.)

Jamie's condition continued to decline, and by January 1993, he was essentially living at the University of Nebraska Medical Center, under the care of Byers W. Shaw, Jr., M. D., one of the nation's leading transplant surgeons. As he waited for a liver, infections were sweeping through Jamie's body, and jaundice had literally turned the young man's skin and eyes yellow – another sure sign of impending liver failure.

Jamie was in his room watching TV when the call finally came. "I have good news for you," said the transplant coordinator. "We found a liver." In a state of shock, Jamie called his dad, who was in New York City preparing to shoot the movie *Quiz Show.* "I woke him up in the middle of the night," recalls Jamie. "He shutdown production and got on a plane."

By 6:00 a. m. the next day, Jamie's liver-transplant surgery was under way. Afterward, he awoke to the human chain formed by his family. The love that encircled him was unforgettable, but so too was the fact that his second chance at life was dependent upon someone else's death – in this case, a 29-year-old man who had suffered a brain aneurysm.

"There's a constant darkness around it," Jamie says of organ donations. "You know that your transplant involves someone else's death." But he has come to accept that "whatever the donor's path in life, their fate isn't tied to yours. It took me a while to recognize that my need for a transplant wasn't going to cause someone else to die."

Initially, Jamie appeared to be making a remarkable recovery. But seven days after the operation, an ultrasound showed a blood clot had formed on the donated organ. Although doctors repaired the liver as best they could, the prognosis wasn't good: It was just a matter of time before the new organ would fail.

Less than two months later, Jamie was back in the hospital full-time waiting for another transplant, again fighting high fevers and rampant infections. Each day his need for another liver grew more critical. "I was really starting to deteriorate," he says. "I had a sense that things were closing in on me."

Among the few bright spots during this desperate period were the visits from his mom and dad. Robert Redford, who had begun directing *Quiz Show* following Jamie's first transplant, told his son, "I can do this movie next year – I can completely shut it down." Jamie declined the offer, not wanting to disrupt the lives of so many people. What Robert Redford did instead speaks volumes about the bond between father and son – and the stalwart determination they share. Every week, after long days of shooting Monday through Saturday afternoon, Redford would catch a flight and be at his son's bedside in Omaha by Saturday evening. The two would spend the weekends watching rough cuts of the film and enjoying each other's company. Come Monday, Redford would fly back. "I really came to rely on this," Jamie recalls.

Jamie's mother, who at the time was completing her Ph. D. in American history, was also a constant presence. Although a dissertation deadline loomed, Lola left New York University, dividing her time between watching over her ailing son and baby-sitting grandson Dylan, while squeezing in work on her doctorate.

As the weeks wore on, Jamie teetered on the edge of total liver failure. If an organ did not become available soon, the outcome would most assuredly be fatal. "I became very anxious," he says. "I really felt like the clock was ticking."

As did Jamie's wife, Kyle, an eighth-grade history teacher. Sitting by her husband's bedside on July 6,

1993, she wished aloud that her birthday – July 7 – would bring with it the ultimate gift: the gift of life for her husband.

Wishes can come true.

The next morning, an exhausted, disheveled transplant coordinator was at Jamie's bedside. "Well, today's your day," he said. The man had just returned from an overnight flight to retrieve a donated liver. This time, the transplant took. The organ, which was donated by the family of a 19-year-old male who died from severe head trauma, functioned well enough for Jamie to be discharged less than two weeks after the operation. Although he will have to take anti rejection medication for the rest of his life, his long-term prognosis is very good.

When he returned home, Jamie wrote letters of gratitude to both donor families. Each word was a struggle. "I told them that I was going to do my best to honor their gift and live my life as well as I could," he says. "I wrote that I hoped they understood they saved a son from growing up without a father, and a loving wife from being a widow."

Two years after the surgery, he established the James Redford Institute for Transplant Awareness, a nonprofit organization dedicated to educating the public about the urgent need for organ and tissue donations and addressing concerns that people have about becoming donors. (More than 60,000 patients nationwide currently await transplants, and it's estimated that each day 12 will die because of a lack of available organs*.)

The institute's most ambitious undertaking is the documentary *The Kindness of Strangers*. Beautifully

*Data as of original publication date.

shot and deeply moving, the film interweaves the stories of four transplant patients with those of two families who donated the organs of lost loved ones. After viewing the film at a Chicago screening, Robert Redford turned to his son and said, "My God, this has to be seen."

Jamie hopes that many people will see *The Kindness of Strangers,* noting that he will never forget the kindness of those strangers who saved his life and forever changed his outlook. "There's not a day that goes by," he says, "that I don't find something to enjoy. My appreciation for the love of my family – my love for my kids – is never far away. The things that really matter, matter that much more."

By Carrie St. Michel
(First printed in Good Housekeeping, September 1999)
Reprinted with permission

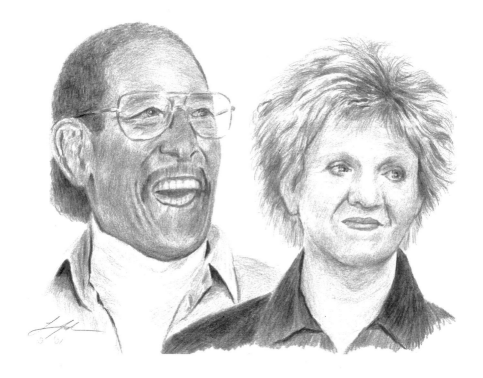

James King
Kidney Recipient

Linda Aadland
Unrelated Kidney Donor

13

A Shared Kidney

The wait for a life-saving organ transplant can be long and excruciating, especially if you have a common blood type and are waiting for a kidney.

The waiting list for kidneys is made up of people from every background and condition, who share a common trait. They are dying and need a transplant to live and have an improved quality of life. Many are on dialysis; some tolerate it better than others. Without a living donor willing to give up a part of his or her body, each must wait for a deceased donor kidney to become available. Dialysis keeps kidney patients alive, but is not a pleasant way to live.

Making it to the top of the waiting list can be like winning the lottery. With luck, you get the next chance to receive a transplant and live a normal life.

For James King, the wait took years. But when he reached the top of the list and was offered a kidney,

James did what most people would never do – he turned it down. When his number came up a second time, he again turned down the offer of a kidney.

Clearly, James is incredibly compassionate. He wanted a transplant, but opted each time to let someone else have the kidney.

"When you have an opportunity to meet people who you are basically competing against for an organ, it is hard to see them going through the ordeals that they are going though," said James. "I wasn't incapacitated by dialysis, so it just seemed right that someone else would have the opportunity, rather than me, at that particular time."

So James twice deferred his opportunity and, each time, the kidney went to someone James had met at dialysis; someone he believed needed it more than he did. Did James worry he would not get a second chance at a normal life?

"I always felt that, when the time came, I would get a kidney and it would work," he said.

Such a heroic stand is not out of the ordinary for James. This was not the first time he had put his life on the line to help others. James proudly defended his country in Vietnam. And, when he returned from Vietnam, he resumed a normal life and raised a family of four children. He lived quietly until polycystic kidney disease robbed him of his health.

With kidney failure, James had to undergo hemodialysis, a process that takes blood from one arm and runs it through a series of filters before returning it to the other arm. Many who must endure dialysis treatments get very sick, some violently so. It is a taxing procedure, but often necessary for those without kidney function. A transplant is the best hope for most patients. Only then can they be freed from the painful ritual of dialysis.

James had to undergo this process several times a week for hours at a time. But James was one of the lucky ones; he tolerated the treatment better than many, so he chose to stay on dialysis and help someone else less fortunate.

Dialysis sessions are routinely scheduled, so patients get to know each other. The misery of the treatment is shared with the company of others in the same situation, all of whom hold a common hope that a kidney will become available so the treatments can stop.

Though James twice turned down that opportunity, the cysts on his kidneys eventually had to be addressed, and both his kidneys were removed. James had to endure life without kidneys for several months until the unexpected happened.

* * *

Driving to work one day, Linda Aadland came up with a most unusual idea: she would donate a kidney. She didn't know anyone who needed a kidney, but she was aware that thousands of people are in need. Organ donation was near to her heart. She had learned about the shortage of organ donors the hard way.

Linda, the mother of three children, had lost her oldest son, Nathan, in an automobile accident in 1995. No one knows what caused the accident; Nate was driving alone when he lost control of the car on a Nebraska road. The car smashed into a tree and burst into flames. Nate never had a chance.

"I feel Nate would have wanted to donate his organs, but it was a fiery crash so we weren't able to harvest them," recalls Linda.

With the loss of her son, Linda became an advocate of organ donation. And, with the memory of her son and his sudden death, Linda contemplated making a gift of life.

"We were always disappointed that we couldn't have donated Nate's organs. And it just came to me in a moment, driving to work one day, that (this) might be a positive thing I could do in his honor."

But when she contacted The Nebraska Medical Center, Linda was told that her donation was not possible. Though the hospital's transplant team wanted to develop an anonymous kidney donor program, it had not done so yet. The surgeons in charge of the kidney transplant program had just recently relocated to Nebraska. They were new to the hospital and had to establish protocols and procedures on how to handle things.

In addition, there was a backlog of traditional kidney transplants from living donors giving to family members, and there were the inevitable transplants of kidneys that suddenly became available from deceased donors. These rather routine transplants would take priority over developing a new, unproven program.

The transplant coordinator took Linda's name and told her they would call her if a program were to be developed. More than a year passed before that call came. In that year, Linda continued to think about donating one of her kidneys, but kept the dream to herself, not even telling her family what she was considering.

After a year of waiting, the Medical Center developed an anonymous kidney donor program. And, after successfully completing the first anonymous transplant, the Transplant Coordinator contacted Linda to see if she was still interested in donating. Despite the passage of time, Linda remained resolute. She wanted to honor her son Nathan by donating a kidney – something she believed he would have wanted to do, had he been able. Yes, she said, she wanted to be tested to see if she could be a kidney donor.

As Linda began the testing, she met with the program's psychologist to make sure she fully understood the ramifications of what she was contemplating. At each step along the way, she was assured that she was under no obligation. If she changed her mind and decided not to proceed, that would be fine.

But Linda never changed her mind. Instead, she grew more and more excited about the prospect of becoming a kidney donor. And when she passed all her testing, she knew this was the right thing for her to do.

Linda was not told who would receive her kidney, but that did not matter. She had learned that there is a kidney shortage and that people died every day for lack of kidney function. She had two kidneys and the testing had proven to her that, most likely, one would be all she ever needed. Linda wanted to give her second kidney away to someone who needed it to live.

* * *

Although James and Linda lived in the same small town of Omaha, Neb., they had never met. They shared a lot of common beliefs and had similar values, but their paths never crossed, not even at The Nebraska Medical Center where they each spent a great deal of time. Linda spent many days there being tested to see if she could donate a kidney. James spent many days there getting prepared for a transplant if a kidney became available.

James and Linda also shared a blood type and had

similar tissue matches. After exhaustive testing for both of them, it was decided that James would be the best candidate to receive Linda's donated kidney. This was the third time James had been offered a life-saving kidney transplant, and it was the first time he would accept this generous offer. His time finally had arrived; he was getting a new kidney. Dialysis soon would be only a memory.

When James received the telephone call that a kidney was available for him, he was quite relieved. Although he continued to tolerate dialysis well, he knew it was time for a transplant.

"It was like a weight had been lifted," James said.

The transplant took place in April 2004. And, to the delight of James and Linda, the kidney worked well.

Three months after surgery, James and Linda met for the first time at Omaha's "Transplant Reunion," an annual gathering of the University's transplant program patients, and an opportunity for patients to meet with each other and share their success stories.

Linda came to the reunion with her husband, but James came alone. Though he knew his children would want to meet his generous donor, he also knew that he risked becoming emotional and didn't want his children to be there if that happened.

James and Linda struck up an immediate friendship.

"We share so many of the same ideas about life, and I feel a strong connection with James," said Linda. Neither could keep from smiling; they looked as though their friendship would be long-lasting.

Non-Directed Donors

It is becoming more common for people to donate kidneys without knowing who the recipient will be. These organs are given to a recipient chosen anonymously by the transplant team. Donor and recipient do not meet until sometime after the transplant – and then only if both agree to meet. These non-directed donations may be called "anonymous," "altruistic" or "stranger" donations.

Paired exchange donations are an extension of non-directed donation. In this situation, two (or more) pairs of donors and recipients are identified, each with incompatible blood types. The kidneys are then swapped – Donor A gives to Recipient B, and Donor B gives to Recipient A. Both donor surgeries take place simultaneously, as do both recipient surgeries.

The first non-directed kidney donations occurred in 1998. Since then, more than 500 non-directed donations have taken place.

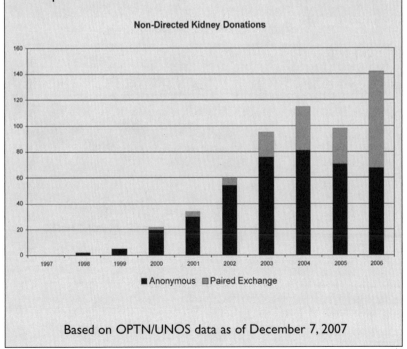

Non-Directed Kidney Donations

Based on OPTN/UNOS data as of December 7, 2007

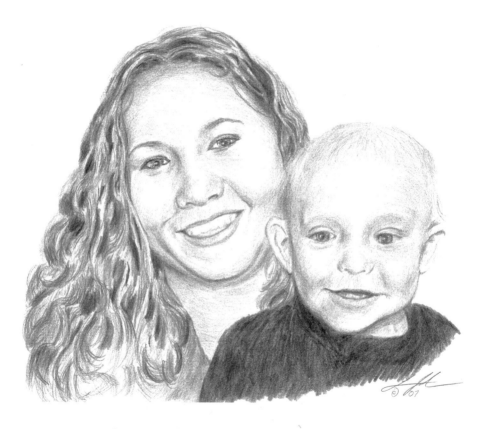

Christa Buettner   **Trey Gulzow**
Liver Donor   **Liver Recipient**

14

'No Way I Wouldn't Help' Nursing Student Is Living Donor For Her Nephew

By Andrea McMaster

A red-and-blue cape embroidered with the Superman logo hangs over his hospital bassinette. Attached to the cape a handwritten note reads, "Christa is my super hero."

Though 7-month-old Trey Gulzow of Lincoln, Neb., didn't yet understand what the word "hero" meant, his hero has allowed him to feel and look like an infant for the first time in his life.

"Trey hardly cried, but you wouldn't blame him if he did," Trey's father, Jeff said. "Adults with their bile backed up like his are often grumpy."

Nearly a 10-pound baby at birth, Trey had appeared in fine shape, but in a few days he grew a bit yellow and wasn't gaining enough weight. A month later, he was diagnosed with biliary atresia, a terminal liver disease. At 6 weeks of age, Trey had surgery to repair his liver, but the surgery failed, and a liver transplant was necessary.

"We had so many emotions. It was a very scary time for the whole family," said Trey's mother, Jackie Gulzow. "But the support was amazing. People came out of the woodwork to help our family."

Instead of waiting for a liver to become available from a deceased donor, Trey's doctors at The Nebraska Medical Center in Omaha suggested living liver donation. Several family members and friends were evaluated to see if they would be a good match.

Trey's aunt, Christa Buettner, a 23-year-old nursing student, was blood compatible and petite, which is good because it was necessary for Trey's donor to be small.

"Anything for my little nephew," Christa said. "If I was a match, there was not even a question in my mind that I would not help Trey."

* * *

Liver regeneration

Living liver donors typically sacrifice one half to three quarters of their liver for a transplant.

"We removed Trey's entire damaged liver, and then replaced it with a portion of Christa's liver – a size which fit in the palm of my hand," explained Debra Sudan, M. D., transplant surgeon at The Nebraska Medical Center and professor of surgery at the University of Nebraska Medical Center.

"The normal size for the liver is about one percent of a person's body mass," Dr. Sudan explained. "That's the target size for the transplant liver in order to optimize early liver function and its ability to regenerate."

Dr. Sudan added that the liver is unique in this trait. "The size increases as much as 100 percent in both donor and recipient, often within six to 12 weeks."

Liver transplants from living donors are a relatively new medical procedure. Although kidneys have been transplanted from living donors since 1954, the first living liver transplant didn't take place until 1989. The operation is becoming more common because the demand for livers far outpaces the number of organs from deceased donors.

* * *

Risks are relatively low

Most living donors are family members – who are most likely to be compatible donors – though unrelated people such as spouses or close friends can also volunteer, as can complete strangers.

In addition to being in good health, donors must undergo a battery of medical tests to ensure their organ is a good match for the recipient.

The Nebraska Medical Center also involves social workers in the evaluation process to ensure the donor is offering the organ for the right reasons. Donors who appear to be coerced or financially compensated are likely to be rejected, and occasionally a psychiatric evaluation may be required before a donor is approved.

For major surgery, the risks for a liver donor are relatively low. The typical operation runs a 10 percent chance of complications and less than 1 percent chance of death, said Dr. Sudan. For the recipient, the most serious complications are rare, but can occur if the new liver does not function properly or if blood vessels develop clots.

"Liver transplant recipients can also develop infections or rejection of the new liver, but these conditions are usually easily controlled with medication," said Dr. Sudan.

"There are significant advantages to receiving an organ from a living donor. The surgery can be planned to occur when the recipient is healthy instead of waiting until the disease is in its advance stages," said Cassandra Smith-Fields, executive director of solid organ transplantation at The Nebraska Medical Center and vice chair of the OPTN/UNOS transplant administrators committee.

"The living donor organs in general function better than deceased donor organs, and a kidney from a living donor transplant may also last longer."

Immediately after the transplant, you could see a difference in little Trey, his mother said.

"His skin was no longer golden, but instead a healthy pink and the whites of his eyes were considerably whiter."

Three weeks post transplant, the Gulzows took Trey home.

"The first day home from the hospital, Trey smiled more than he ever had," his father said. "He also rolled over for the first time. Before, his large, bloated, fluid-filled stomach kept him from being physically active."

Trey Gulzow celebrated his first birthday Dec. 12. He now is as active as any young toddler.

"One day, he'll understand what his hero, Christa, did for him," said Jackie. "He'll also understand why everyone we meet calls him a superhero too."

For now, though, it's enough that Trey can fall

asleep each night at home underneath his Superman sheets, next to a mural of the Man of Steel on his nursery wall.

By Andrea McMaster, media consultant at
The Nebraska Medical Center
(Article originally appeared in the March-April issue of the Update, the bimonthly magazine of the United Network of Organ Sharing.)

Reprinted by permission.

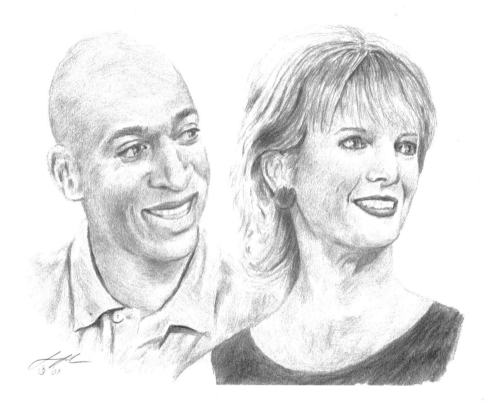

Will Smith
Kidney Recipient

Ellen Souvinoy
Kidney Donor

15

He Saved Her Life, She Saved His

Ellen Souviney's position was not unusual. In her mid-40s, she suddenly began to gain weight. She chalked it up to getting older, but having an excuse for putting on the weight was not sufficient.

"I had never been overweight and then, suddenly, all this weight piled on when I hit middle age," said Ellen. She wanted to do something about it.

She sought the help of Will Smith, a personal trainer who had helped her husband get into shape. Will was confident he could help Ellen, but this would be more than a physical challenge. Ellen's weight gain was accompanied by low self-esteem.

"When Ellen first started coming to me, she was a physical wreck. She was very much overweight, (with) low self-esteem. And I told Ellen she could easily be a size four, if she just put her mind to it," said Will.

Ellen just laughed at Will's suggestion. She was a

size sixteen and had a hard time believing such a drastic change was possible.

Will knew a lot about getting into shape, and his knowledge was backed up by his own experience. A champion body builder, he had once held the titles of "Mr. Europe" and "Mr. Italy."

Will and Ellen began working out together. With his help, Ellen lost an astounding 55 pounds, going from a size 16 dress down to a 2. Perhaps more importantly though, she regained the self-confidence she had lost.

But as Ellen was getting into shape and her health was improving, she could not help but notice that Will's health was failing. Will suffered from kidney failure brought on by an infection that had gone untreated. He required dialysis three times a week and did not tolerate the treatments well.

Will described his condition: "I had complete renal failure; there was no kidney function whatsoever. I had to be on dialysis three, four times a week because of my size and I would sit there five hours a day being connected to a machine to have my blood cleaned."

Will Smith's health continued to decline, and perilously so. His health was so poor that the simplest of tasks were a challenge. The champion body builder had problems spotting his clients in weight lifting and could barely take his children out to enjoy ice cream.

"It was grim. You hold on to faith and you believe. I had one doctor tell me, 'Maybe you have five years.' Others were a little more optimistic, but I would always hear the negative comments. That stayed in my head. You think, 'I only have little time left.'"

Several family members wanted to help. Each got tested to determine if they could give Will a kidney. Unfortunately, none was a close enough match.

Friends and acquaintances also offered to be tested,

but Will discouraged them from going forward, thinking that donating a kidney would be too much to ask of anyone.

Ellen too, offered to donate a kidney, but Will offered no encouragement. Will is African-American; Ellen is Caucasian. Will is male; Ellen is female. Because Will thought a match was unlikely, he didn't take her offer seriously at first.

"(My husband and I) cared a lot about him and his health," said Ellen. "I really felt like Will had saved my life." She wanted to see if she could save his.

Determined, Ellen researched kidney donation on the Internet. For every excuse Will proffered, she found the facts to back up the opposing opinion. She was resolved to follow through with her plan, or find a reason it could not be done.

Will finally agreed to allow the testing to see if Ellen was a match. But he remained skeptical of Ellen's offer.

"It was hard to understand why someone who had no ties with you would want to come up and give part of themselves," said Will. "I didn't want to believe it. I fought it. I kept telling her, 'No, no, no.' And every time I argued, Ellen would come back through her research. Finally, when she convinced me, I think I said yes just to get her off my back, not thinking she would match me."

Much to Will's surprise, Ellen turned out to be a suitable match. More importantly, she was prepared to go through with the operation and give Will a chance at a better life.

On October 2, 2001, Ellen donated her kidney to Will. The man who had given Ellen a new life by helping her get in shape got his own life back again with the gift of a kidney.

How does Will feel about his new lease on life?

"I feel like Superman, to be honest with you," he said.

Ellen was amazed that 'such a little thing' could mean so much to Will.

The kidney is not the only thing the two have in common; each credits the other for making a difference in his or her life.

Ellen realized that, with Will's help, her life would be years longer and much healthier, "I really felt like he had saved my life. There is no way to repay that," she said.

And Will credits Ellen for the improvement in his life. "It's a new life, a new experience," he said. "(Before the transplant), I could not pick up my infant son. Now he's seven and weighs 82 pounds, and I can pick him up with no problem."

Biological Relationship

As anti-rejection medication gets better, a biological relationship between donor and recipient is becoming less important. Instead, other relationships, such as the strong emotional bond between spouses or in-laws, or even a more casual relationship between friends or co-workers, may prompt people to donate. Sometimes, in an anonymous or paired exchange donation, a donor gives an organ without knowing who will receive it.

As recently as 1991, more than 90 percent of donors were biologically related to their recipients. In 2007, more than two in five had no biological relationship.

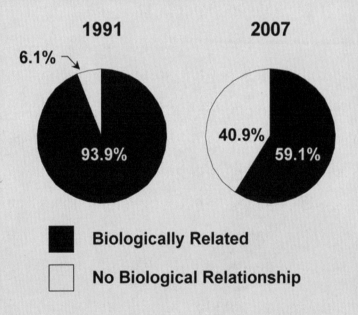

1991

6.1%

93.9%

2007

40.9%   59.1%

■ **Biologically Related**

☐ **No Biological Relationship**

Based on OPTN/UNOS data as of December 7, 2007

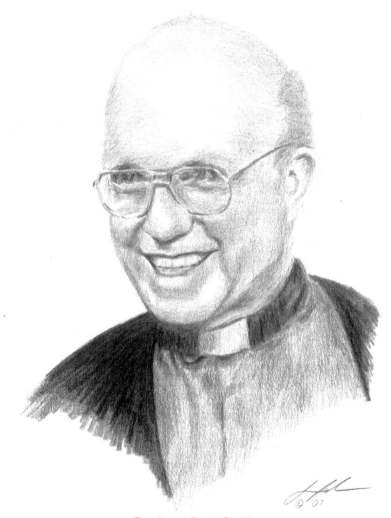

Father Pat Sullivan
Anonymous Kidney Donor

16

Where Is Father Pat's Kidney?

It was just an article in the *New York Times Sunday Magazine,* but it changed the life of Father Pat, a Catholic priest. He was upset by what he read but, more importantly, he was moved to take action. He wanted to do what he could do to eliminate an injustice by some who were taking advantage of those trapped in poverty.

The article, written by Michael Finkel, was about the buying and selling of kidneys. The facts were alarming. With more than 50,000* people in need of a life-saving kidney transplant, too few people were willing to help. There was (and still is) a critical shortage of organs available for transplantation.

Some kidney patients receive organs from deceased donors– normally people who have been declared brain dead due to accident or injury. Others have received kidneys donated by family members. But the demand

*Data as of original publication date.

for kidneys far outweighs the supply, and several thousand people die each year waiting for a kidney.

In desperation, a few who needed a life-saving kidney transplant had turned to the black market. The cost was high, both financially and morally. Only those with substantial financial resources could afford the price of a black-market kidney. This practice is illegal in the United States and throughout most of the world. Still, with enough money, a broker could assemble the deal. The recipient would fly to a foreign country – often India or Turkey – where the operation would take place. The kidney donor – or more accurately, the kidney seller – was often a person with few choices but to sell part of his body to earn money needed to help support his family.

What would drive a person to leave the United States, with the best health care system in the world, to receive a kidney transplant in a foreign country? The transplants often are performed in less-than-ideal conditions and some recipients have died from the surgery. Others contracted dreaded diseases like hepatitis from contaminated instruments. Kidney sellers often are not properly screened to determine if they are healthy enough to donate. And the follow-up? It can be nonexistent, as might be expected for an illegal surgical procedure. Why would anyone risk this?

The answer is simple: Of the thousands of people on the transplant wait list, almost two-thirds are waiting for kidneys. Some of those patients simply are not willing to take the risk of waiting, and money is a powerful incentive to those so desperately poor that they have few alternatives. On the black market, the rich would receive a transplant and the poor would receive needed cash. It is a classic case of those with means taking advantage of those in need.

For 30 years, Fr. Pat carried a signed donor card witnessed by two others. It was testimony to his desire to donate any needed organs or tissue in the event of his death.

"I figured, why not? I can save someone's life by giving away what I no longer need," said Fr. Pat.

Studies have shown that most people are willing to donate their organs after death. Unfortunately, not many are able to do so. Sickness, old age or cause of death each can rob a person of the ability to be an organ donor. Most people who die simply do not have organs suitable for transplantation.

The science of organ transplantation has evolved over the years. New drugs improve the chances of successful transplantation. Genetic matches are becoming less important. It is no longer necessary to be related biologically to be considered a candidate for organ donation. Donations from friends, spouses and strangers are becoming more common. With this knowledge, Fr. Pat wondered if he could donate one of his kidneys to someone who needed it.

"It is hard to be a Franciscan for 38 years and a priest for 30 years without something sinking in. I was faced with some alarming facts about the selling of donor organs and the number of people who die while waiting for transplants," said Father Pat. "It seems that God has blessed us with an over-capacity as far as the kidneys are concerned. When one is removed, the other quickly takes up the slack, grows a bit and does the whole job quite nicely."

Prior to reading the *New York Times* article, Fr. Pat never considered becoming a living kidney donor. But now, for the first time in his life, he considered making the gift of life. Although he did not know anyone personally who needed a transplant, he thought this was something that he could do.

Two things about Fr. Pat's gift – if he were selected as a kidney donor – would be somewhat unique. The first is that he would not direct that his kidney be given to anyone in particular. Rather, he would rely on the transplant committee to choose the recipient based on need and genetic match. The second is that his decision to donate was very much motivated by his religious faith.

As a Catholic priest, Fr. Pat always tried to follow the teachings of Jesus. It seemed that a kidney donation would be a good response to Jesus' invitation to "love one another." Fr. Pat could be a "Good Samaritan" and do unto others as he would want done to himself if he needed a kidney. At 56 years of age, he was approaching the age where he might soon exceed the limits imposed by some transplant centers.

Fr. Pat began to research kidney transplants. He spoke to and read firsthand accounts of others who were donors to see what the process was really like. He went to Websites where organ donors, potential donors and others chatted about organ donation.

His research convinced him that live kidney donation is increasingly common and that it has become rather safe, with no known long-term effects to the donor. The research confirmed for him that donating a kidney was something he wanted to do.

"Even well-educated people often don't understand that a healthy person can give a kidney and go on with a perfectly normal life," said Fr. Pat. "Complications, of course, are possible but are not frequent. My surgeon told me that, statistically, kidney donation has about the same risk factor as getting a hernia repair operation."

Fr. Pat contacted a transplant center and explained

his desire to become a donor. The transplant team gathered his data and helped him to begin the process. The testing consisted of physical tests, mental tests and a thorough review of his medical history.

A doctor, a nurse, a social worker and a psychologist interviewed him. They had to make sure he knew what he was getting into and that he was more or less sane. They would look for ulterior motives and hidden agendas. Ironically, it is through the psychological examination that the staff may learn the "donor" is not really a donor at all. Some have been caught trying to sell the kidney, while others feel pressured from family members to donate. Neither of these could be the case for Fr. Pat – he did not have a specific recipient in mind.

The surgical staff had to assure that he was physically healthy enough to be a donor. Ethically, they would not subject a donor to surgery if there were any likelihood that it would cause harm. The liability of running any such risk would not be worth it. Saving one life is not worth the cost of losing another.

The testing, Fr. Pat found, is extensive. Many blood samples are taken for various testing purposes. And urine tests are common – including one test where the potential donor collects 24 hours worth of urine in a plastic bottle – a test much easier on males than on females. The collected urine must be kept cold. (There is nothing like warm urine gone bad.)

Finally, Fr. Pat was accepted as a donor. Since his was to be a non-directed donation, the team had the luxury of being able to compare his blood chemistry with many of the people on the waiting list to determine the best possible match. He could be matched with the person they determined to be least likely to reject the kidney.

For a non-directed kidney donation, great lengths

are taken to maintain the confidentiality of both the donor and the recipient. Neither knows the other, and the recipient may not even know if the kidney comes from a living donor or a deceased person. While the surgeries are underway, donor and recipient family members stay in separate areas to prevent them from accidentally meeting during the hours of waiting.

As Fr. Pat said, "It's sort of like when you give blood: you never know who got your blood and the recipient never knows where the blood came from. This, of course, fits nicely with what Jesus taught: 'When you give alms, don't even let your left hand know what your right hand is doing.'"

Fr. Pat understood the risks and was willing to accept them. A recipient was identified and a date for surgery was set.

There are two basic methods for removing a kidney. The first is the open procedure, where the surgeon makes an incision eight to 10 inches long just below the ribs from the front to the back. The other type of surgery is laparoscopic, where three very small incisions are made and the kidney is removed through a fourth somewhat larger incision about three to four inches long. The longer incision is just large enough for the kidney and the surgeon's hand.

Fr. Pat's surgeon preferred the older, open method. Although this method requires more healing time, it allows the surgeon more room to perform the surgery and more chance of immediately spotting and correcting any surgical mistakes.

Fr. Pat arrived as scheduled for his surgical procedure, having prepared by cleaning out his system inside and out. He had eaten no solid food since breakfast the day before and had chugged a bottle of laxatives to thoroughly empty his bowels. He was ready.

He checked in and went to the pre-op area, where he changed into a gown. He was hooked up with an intravenous fluid and the transplant coordinator asked him if he was certain he wanted to go through with the surgery, giving him one last chance to change his mind. Although he appreciated the offer, Fr. Pat was comfortable with his decision. He would donate a kidney. With that, he was given a shot of anesthetic to relax him. The shot is the last thing Fr. Pat remembers prior to surgery. The surgery was uneventful and went well for both parties.

After surgery, Fr. Pat was moved to one floor for recuperation, while the recipient was moved to another floor. This is done partially for anonymity and partially for safety. Often, donors and recipients are family members and have the same last name. With donors and recipients on different floors, the nursing staff is less likely to make a mistake with medication.

As with the recovery from any extensive surgery, patients are encouraged to get out of bed and walk a bit whenever they can. Even a short walk allows the blood to circulate a little more and exercises the muscles. That is another reason to keep the donors and recipients on different floors. Casual conversation between two patients walking the hallway can destroy anonymity.

Although Fr. Pat had been through a battery of tests and had done his homework about the donation process, he encountered one surprise – the deep emotional impact of the donation. It was easy for him to describe the surgery from a physical standpoint. He could easily talk about the testing, his physical well being and what was going on inside his body. But he was unprepared for what was happening to him emotionally.

The first time he was overcome by the emotion of what he had done occurred soon after being released from the hospital. He had learned that walking made him more comfortable and he walked often. When he awoke in the middle of the night to go to the bathroom, he decided to take a short walk prior to going back to bed. Catching a glimpse of the get-well cards and balloons sent by friends and family triggered an emotional reaction he had not expected.

Fr. Pat began crying uncontrollably. The tears were not from sadness, but rather from emotion surrounding the enormity of what he had done. He was able to give life to another through his donation of a kidney. In return, he received wonderful expressions of personal and professional care. And, most importantly, he had survived it all. Donating the kidney was a remarkable achievement that affected him deeply. Fr. Pat did not know why he was crying, but the outburst lasted about 10 minutes, through half a box of tissues.

A second time emotions got the better of him was when he returned to the altar to say Mass. One week to the day after surgery, Fr. Pat was back serving his parish. Most of those present were aware of his surgery and had been praying for both him and the recipient. He became entirely choked up when he repeated the words he had said so many times, "Take this body which is given for you. Drink, this is my blood which is shed for you."

As the Bible says, "God is love." And Fr. Pat adds, "As an act of love, organ donation can be an experience from God...I would encourage potential donors not to be afraid to get in touch with their spiritual roots. They are the source of strength that we all need."

Fr. Pat has never met his kidney recipient. He continues to respect the confidentiality of his generous donation. Unless the recipient or his/her family seeks to find out who donated the kidney, the two will not meet.

The recipient sent a lovely thank-you note, unsigned, through the surgeon, but has opted to remain anonymous, which is fine with Fr. Pat. He's also comfortable with meeting if the recipient ever decides to do so.

About the anonymity, Fr. Pat becomes philosophical. "The advantage of not meeting is that I can imagine, if I wish, that my recipient will now go on to win the Nobel Prize, be elected President, and find a cure for cancer and the common cold. What if I met him/her and he/she turned out to be the head of a neo-Nazi biker gang, grateful for another chance to wipe out all inferior races? Do I ask for my kidney back? So, either meeting or not meeting has its own advantages and disadvantages."

Much time has passed since Fr. Pat donated his kidney and he remains an advocate for organ transplantation. He writes and speaks to others who are considering this unselfish gift, and he tries to help them arrive at a decision that is right for them. Although he would never try to talk someone into donating, he hopes more people will at least consider organ donation. Some will do it during their lives as a living donor; others will do it postmortem as deceased donors.

For those who join the club of living organ donors, Fr. Pat offers these words of encouragement: "Don't be afraid to savor what you have done and give yourself a pat on the back! You know you did a beautiful thing that you can treasure in this life and in eternity. You can honestly and humbly face the reality of times of depression, and at the same time not let it dim the happiness of having done a really beautiful thing for someone."

Father Pat can be contacted by email:
PSofmcap@aol.com

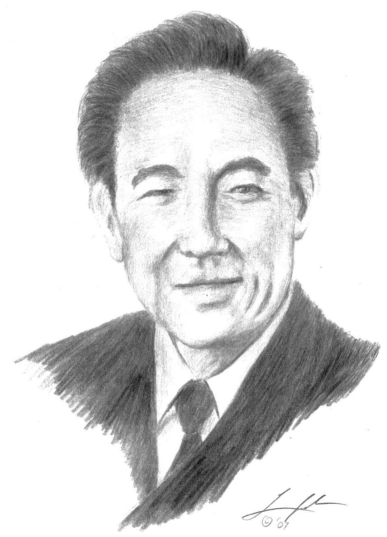

Dr. Kenneth Moritsugu
Donor Family

17

Making The Right Choice – Twice

By Dr. Kenneth Moritsugu

Over the past four years, it has been my privilege to represent donor families everywhere, at this National Donor Recognition Program – a ceremony, solemn as well as joyful, to acknowledge the many heroes of our country who made the ultimate humanitarian gesture of organ and tissue donation.

"We celebrate Life, the Gift of Life, the Circle of Life: the circle that has no beginning and no end; the circle that includes the many true heroes of transplantation:

- ◆ Heroes, like the transplant candidates, who anxiously and patiently wait with hope for their transplant, that a miracle will happen;
- ◆ Heroes, like the transplant recipients, those brave ones who placed their faith and trust in the science and skill of the health professionals, and who show every day by their lives that transplantation works;

- Heroes, like their families, who provide the love and support for these individuals during their wait, and during and after their transplant;
- Heroes, like the transplant professionals, who with their knowledge and skill help bring together the various forces and resources to help the miracle of transplantation happen – and especially today,
- Heroes, like the donors, both living and dead, who gave so unselfishly of themselves, as the ultimate gesture of human generosity, to make the miracle of transplantation possible, without whom no miracle could happen;
- And heroes, like the donor families who <u>assured</u> that this could happen, often in times of deepest tragedy and sorrow – the survivors, who, despite our losses and our grief, continue our struggle to go on with our lives.

The Gift of Life is about people who care, at every level, without whom nothing could happen – because donation and transplantation is not a sterile medical process, but a personal, human deed, which touches people, closely, personally, intimately – through which another human receives a new lease on life; an enhanced quality of living; a new outlook on humanity.

Donor families each have their stories. Each story is different, each story is special. But what is common to all, is the uncommon generosity of the human spirit, often in time of grief and tragedy, to rise above personal self-concern, to help others in need of transplantation, in need of life, through the ultimate gifts of the donors, *their* ultimate acts of human kindness.

Through their generosity, in their brief moments on this earth, these donors whom we acknowledge today, donors everywhere, have achieved greatness – ordinary people, who have made extraordinary things happen.

Donors and donor families, without whom the miracles of transplantation could not occur at all.

Each of us has our own story; and I am no different. Permit me to share my story with you.

Five years ago, my late wife, Donna Lee, was in a severe auto accident and was soon brain dead. And because she and I had talked long before about what each of us wanted when we died, she became an organ and tissue donor. I *had* the *privilege of carrying out* her *wishes*.

And because of that decision, five years ago:
- A police detective in Tampa Florida, received a new heart;
- A young diabetic hospital custodian in Washington, DC, received a pancreas and a kidney;
- A 12-year-old child, who was on dialysis and failing in school, received the other kidney. He is now making straight A's, and is on his way to college;
- A retired schoolteacher in Pennsylvania received a new liver; and was able to spend Christmas again with her three children;
- A young retarded woman in Baltimore, MD, received one cornea; and the other cornea provided a new vision to a 49 year old local government worker.

Donna Lee was simply an ordinary person, who accomplished extraordinary things. Without her generosity, as well as those of so many other donors, this would never have been possible.

But that is not the end of the story.

Seven months ago, my younger daughter, Vikki Lianne, only 22 years old, was struck by an auto while crossing a street. She suffered massive brain injury, and died after three days. We believed she would have wanted to be an organ donor, and so we made those arrangements.

Later, my older daughter, Erika, said to me, "Dad, you did the right thing." Because, unbeknownst to me, after Donna Lee died, my two daughters had had several discussions about their *own* lives. And they noted how so many others had benefited from Donna's ultimate/final gift, how we the family had derived such comfort in our loss.

And Vikki had stated that she too, wanted to be an organ donor. It was, in her words, the least she could do for fellow humanity.

I cannot describe to you how proud I feel, about the character and the generosity of my children, of all donors and donor families everywhere.

Out of the mouths of our younger generation. At that time, they were both just emerging from their teens. If these young people can be so altruistic and humanitarian, why can we all not be so, as well?

And because of Vikki:

- A mother of five children from upstate New York received her heart and a new lease on life for herself and for her family;
- A widow with four children received her lung;
- A 59 year old man from Washington, DC, an active volunteer with a charitable organization in the area, received her liver;
- A widower with one daughter received one kidney;
- A married working father of several children received the other kidney.
- A 26 year old man in Florida received one cornea, and a 60 year old woman in Pennsylvania received the other.

I was privileged to be part of THEIR decision, their generosity, their gift of life, their ultimate gesture of humanity, just as all donor families are part of their loved ones generosity.

Because of Donna Lee, and because of Vikki Lianne, and because of so many other organ and tissue donors, many other people have directly gained, from a renewed life, and an improved quality of life.

But when one hears of organ and tissue donation and transplantation, there is an immediate sense that this is an issue that affects only a small number of the public.

Nothing can be farther from the truth.

Like a pebble tossed into a pond, the ripples of life expand outward, affecting not just the donors and recipients, but families, friends, colleagues, coworkers, and others; and in turn these affect so many others, in ever-expanding Circles of Life.

These other individuals, but for the miracle of donation and transplantation, the Gift of Life, would have lost a parent, a friend, a colleague, to death and disability. Donation and transplantation affect society broadly, not just one person.

Ordinary people, performing extraordinary deeds.

And these stories abound – heroes all. Each of us has a special story! If only we could better get these stories before the public.

AND WE CAN! As living donors, and as donor families, we have a credibility unmatched by any other, because we have been through it all ourselves, and can speak from personal experience.

Many recipients are with us today, many coming from a distance, to give thanks for the gifts of America's donors. We congratulate you and embrace you, because we see in your lives that TRANSPLANTATION WORKS!

Today, we remember the donors, our loved ones, for who they were, for what they did, and for their ultimate gestures of human generosity. Ordinary people, who have accomplished extraordinary deeds – America's true heroes.

By Dr. Kenneth Moritsugu, Deputy Surgeon General
(*Transcript of speech given at National Donor Recognition Ceremony, April 13, 1997.*)
Reprinted by Permission

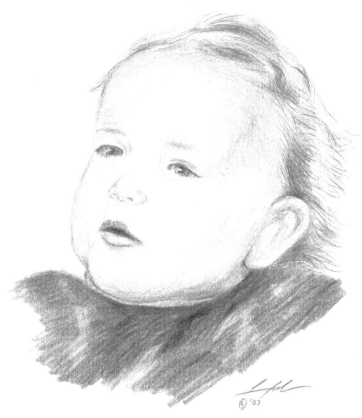

Ellis Joshua Bergstrom
Heart Recipient

18

You Taught Me About Love

By Sam Bergstrom (Ellis' Father)

Monday, December 18, 2006 2:39 PM CST

Dear Ellis,

I have often daydreamed of a time when I would have the opportunity to tell your story to a large group of people. Maybe this would be at your wedding reception, high school graduation or some other event where people are talking about how special you are. I actually pictured me telling your story to you in a time when you needed some encouragement, like when you didn't make the high school baseball team or didn't get a lead role in the school play. I imagined me telling you your own story to remind you of how special, brave and inspiring you are. So here is your story:

I remember the day you were born – a rainy and stormy day in March. Maybe the heavens were telling me what I was in store for. Anyway, I remember how I felt when you entered the world. I remember feeling like I just met this squishy-faced kid and I already loved him beyond words. Your Mom and I didn't really get to do the normal "hang out in the room with your new baby" stuff because you were sick. By the time the doctors figured out what was wrong, you weren't just sick, but as sick as a baby can get. We knew that parenthood would be full of worry and gray hair, but give us a break – you were only one day old. They told us they had to do a procedure immediately to fix your heart and said they weren't sure you would survive. Well, you did survive.

We then spent some time in the hospital with you hoping we could take you home soon. They then told us that the only chance of this would be a heart surgery to fix your drum. The doctors told us again that they weren't sure you would be able to survive. The surgeon even asked if you were baptized yet. You were the night before. Again, Ellis, the rock star, did great and survived.

A few weeks later, the doctors did a silly test on your brain and told us that you were very sick. They said you would never be able to do all the stuff you love to do like talk, walk, read books and give hugs. The only sad part of this is that we had learned nothing from you before and we actually believed them. You showed all of us.

While we were still in the hospital, you were sick in other parts too. Your liver, kidneys, lungs and heart all were doing their best to work. The doctors again told us that we would never be able to bring you home. We were with you every day and tried to make you comfortable by not letting people do stuff to you. Once again, you proved everyone wrong and you got better. You survived and we got to finally bring you home.

We thought our time together would be short because you needed a new heart and they didn't want to give you one because of the stuff they told us about your brain. Before we knew it, you were playing with toys, saying "Mama" and "Dada," blowing kisses, and walking in your walker. The doctors were blown away and told us you would get your new heart.

After you got your new heart, the doctors again said that you would struggle to breathe and would not be able to do it on your own. Well, once again, you did it and proved them wrong.

We have all learned from your story that you are brave and a survivor. We also thought that if you fought so hard every step of the way and proved everyone wrong, you would continue to do the same for a long, long time. I'm here to say that you didn't have to keep fighting. It's okay to say, "I'm tired and want to rest." We are so proud of you. We are so proud to be your mama and dada.

It's amazing how much someone can learn from a two-year-old. It's even more amazing how much I have learned from you. You have taught me a lifetime of lessons in two-and-a-half short years.

You taught me to stop and smell the roses. You showed me this by taking your time and examining things most of us don't even see. You had no problem with all of a sudden stopping in the middle of the parking lot on the way to a therapy appointment, sitting down, then patting the ground, telling us to sit down next to you to look at rocks.

You taught me how important determination and will are. One doctor said that you would never walk. Then at a therapy appointment, while you were actually walking in your walker, another doctor said, "Hey, this kid shouldn't be able to walk." It doesn't matter what people say or even what your body says. What matters is, what does your will say?

You taught me about your mom. You taught me that the woman I married turned out to be the most wonderful mother in the world. We both lucked out on this one.

You taught me life is good. Despite spending a quarter of your life in the hospital and being poked by hundreds of needles, you always seemed to get excited about something or have a smile on your face (when you were at home anyway). Life is good. Life is worth enduring the pain to get to the good stuff.

You taught me about love. Before you came along, I had no idea I was capable of feeling so much love. The crazy part is that the love grows more each and everyday. I thought this was impossible. But just like all of your impossible obstacles... anything is possible.

Every morning before I would leave for work, I would peek my head in your room and thank God for you and your Mother. I will continue to peek my head in your room and thank God for every minute we spent together, all of the wonderful memories, and all of the lessons you taught me by just being Ellis.

We will always love you and miss you more than you can ever know.

Love,

Dada

Written by Sam Bergstrom, Ellis' Father
(First posted on caringbridge. org)
Reprinted by permission

http://www.caringbridge.org/mn/ellis/

*To the Glory of God and
in Celebration of the Life of
Ellis Joshua Bergstrom*

*Born March 25, 2004
Died December 4, 2006*

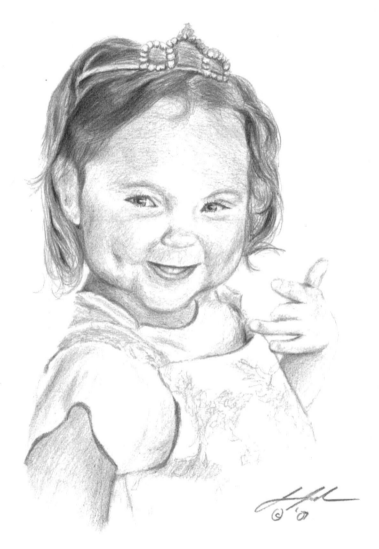

Lili Whitaker
Kidney Recipient

19

Lili Keeps On Blooming

Julie Newland had just moved back to Lansing, Michigan, where she had attended Michigan State a few years earlier. She was returning with the hope of getting her teaching certificate. Just as her life was beginning to take shape, she received some unexpected news.

It was August 2002 and Julie learned that she was pregnant. She had been dating Bruce Whitaker for only about five months, and the news had come as an unexpected surprise. Although she had hoped to start a family some day, Julie was not ready to start yet. The reality was she was single and pregnant. She had some tough decisions to make.

Although the pregnancy was unplanned, Julie wanted to keep the baby. She thought, "I'm 30 years old. I'm responsible. I'm pregnant and I have to keep it." Bruce reluctantly agreed. Though neither was ready to become a parent, both would deal with the hand God had given them.

The pregnancy was progressing smoothly when, a few days after her 20-week ultrasound, Julie received a letter from the Health Department asking her to repeat the test. She was not alarmed. She dealt with the Health Department often and thought, "They screw up things all the time." The need for a second ultrasound was unclear. The letter said it was because of the baby's position, which sounded reasonable enough.

As Julie was having the retest, she began chatting with the technician and learned that the technician was looking for the baby's kidneys, which had not shown up during the first test. This casual conversation was the first time Julie had any indication that something might be wrong with her baby.

During the retest, neither the technician nor the radiologist, whom the technician called in, were able to identify the kidneys. Further, the radiologist was concerned about the dangerously low level of amniotic fluid.

The radiologist recommended going to a level two ultrasound, and would send a letter to Julie's doctor to approve the test. Only then would the procedure be scheduled. Julie's baby was in trouble, however, and she decided she could not wait for the Health Department bureaucracy to weed its way through paperwork.

Fortunately, there was another option. Bruce contacted Dr. Petroff, one of his Michigan State professors, who took a personal interest. Pulling some strings, Dr. Petroff got the ultrasound scheduled in three weeks. Until then, Julie was put on bed rest.

The wait was long and excruciating, but it was better than what would have happened without the connection. Julie's level two ultrasound provided answers, but not the ones the couple had expected or prayed for.

The baby, a girl, had no kidneys.

Clearly, Julie was facing some tough choices. To terminate the pregnancy would require proof the baby could not survive. More tests were needed to determine her viability.

The first test, an MRI, required that the baby be anesthetized. Julie was given a local to dull the pain of her injection. Then the needle was inserted through her abdomen into the baby's leg. The needle stick must have hurt badly as the little girl began to kick wildly. Julie felt so sorry for the pain her baby was enduring. An outside force had penetrated the comfort of the womb, but the baby was proving she was a fighter.

For nearly an hour Julie had to lie still, unable to see anything but the painted metal machine that entombed her. It was a horrible experience. All Julie could think of were her guardian angels that would help her endure this torture. And to make matters worse, the baby kept moving. Julie worried that the test would not be as clear as needed and would have to be repeated.

The MRI was expected to prove the baby had no kidneys, but such was not the case. The test results added more confusion to an already confusing situation. There was urine in the baby's bladder, and some more urine was excreted during the test. The urine had to be coming from somewhere. As they examined the baby further, they found renal tissue on her right side. The kidney was not formed as well as would be expected for a child of this gestation, but clearly there was enough tissue to produce the urine.

Julie decided not to terminate the pregnancy. There was a chance, although slim, that the baby could survive. She searched online with others who had faced such difficult decisions. Most of those she contacted who had carried to term were very happy that they did.

It would be difficult for Julie, but she would carry the baby for as long as God would allow her to do so.

Still concerned about the lack of amniotic fluid and its effect on the baby's health, medical professionals recommended other testing to check lung function. The test, although not 100 percent accurate, would likely provide more information about the baby and her chances for survival. When the results came back, there was more bad news. It appeared the baby's lungs would not be able to function.

Julie's faith was being tested yet again. By now she had become quite accustomed to talking with God. In the beginning she asked, "Why me?" Before long, she stopped asking why and began asking for God's help. This simple act began to transform her prayers. Julie soon was thanking God for her many blessings, concentrating on the positive rather than the negative. Instead of being angry at her situation, she became grateful for her many blessings. She would need God's help to get through this difficult time.

Although another test could provide more information about the baby's lung function, it posed a serious threat to the already ailing baby. The test could have killed the baby, and that was a risk this mother was not willing to take. The best option appeared to be to let nature take its course. Julie put her life and that of her baby into the hands of God. She would carry the baby to term even though the chances of her baby's survival were small.

Soon Julie came to accept that her baby would not survive. She hoped for the best, but planned for the worst, even preparing for her baby's funeral. She wanted to honor the child within her, and make her life as good as possible. Whether the baby died in the womb, or shortly after birth, Julie would do whatever she could for her baby. She wanted nothing more than for her child to have a quality life regardless of how short it would inevitably be.

As Julie's due date approached, she met with the medical staff and the neonatal doctor to determine the best course of action. They wanted desperately to beat the odds, no matter how unlikely. The baby was in a very delicate state, and one thing was abundantly clear: The baby would not survive long after birth without help. The best chance of survival would be to induce labor so the entire neonatal team could be present to take action.

Unfortunately, things do not always go as planned, and Julie's baby did not agree with the schedule. Before labor was induced, the baby decided it was time to leave the comfort of her womb. She was going to enter the world on her own terms.

The labor was intense, but relatively quick. There was no time to have either the mother or the baby hooked up to monitors. The baby was on the way out, ready or not.

Julie wanted desperately for the ordeal to end. She had spent so much time wondering about her baby's health, that she just wanted to get through the delivery. She needed to meet her baby, and the baby needed to meet her Mom. The baby girl, who would be named Lili, was born at 6:59. The neonatal team had expected problems with the baby's lungs, but was pleasantly surprised when she was born screaming. Lili's lungs seemed fine. They put her on oxygen as a precaution and began examining her immediately.

They expected that the baby would be deformed,

and they were wrong here too. She was beautiful. She had 10 fingers and 10 toes. There was nothing unusual except that she cried louder than they had thought she could. Everything seemed absolutely normal.

As Lili quickly underwent numerous tests, she continued to amaze the neonatal staff and the young mother. She was doing great. Finally, the tests were concluded and Julie was able to hold Lili for the first time.

Julie could not believe her good fortune. Her baby had a difficult fight ahead – but the child was a fighter.

Family members from both sides continued to gather and learn the good news that the baby had been born alive. Given the pregnancy's circumstances, a priest was brought in very soon after birth to baptize the child. All the family members were allowed in the room to witness the ceremony, which, though wonderful, was also very emotional as everyone knew Lili could give up her struggle at any moment. But Lili refused to surrender.

Julie had feared losing her child but, within 24 hours, was instead taking her home. Lili was not out of danger, but she was alive and fighting to stay that way.

Julie had done such a good job of preparing for the worst that she was not prepared for the best. She had planned a funeral, but had not planned a life. She was not ready to give the baby the special care she would require. All she could do was make her comfortable and give her love.

Friends and family members came by to meet the baby, to bring gifts and to help. The visitors' kindness and generosity were enormously helpful and the new mother was grateful beyond words.

Within a few days, however, Lili was having problems and needed help. Going back to the hospital now was the scariest thing Julie could imagine. Of course she was not ready to let her baby die, but the hospital could not provide the quality of life she wanted for her baby.

Julie agonized over the decision. Her baby's quality of life was so important to her, and she knew she could give her the love she deserved at home. She was not sure Lili would get the same level of love in the cold hospital setting, even if that meant a longer life.

Julie did know this: If Lili were in the hospital, Julie would be there with her. Her life would be on hold as long as her baby could hold on.

Julie trusted in God's plan, not knowing what it was. Did He want Lili to survive, or to die comfortably at home? There were no easy answers; she had accepted the reality that she would lose her baby.

In the end, Julie agreed Lili's best chances would be in the hospital, even though the experience Lili had there was excruciating. Only nine days old, Lili was returning to the hospital with no certainty of ever coming home again. It was too much for Julie to bear. She cried all day long.

Lili took well to her new surroundings and began eating well. The constant blood draws were difficult, but Lili handled her testing better than Julie did. Julie could not stand to see her baby poked. Lili was not a fan of it, either, but she soon got used to it.

Eventually Julie had to get a room at the Ronald McDonald House across the street from the hospital. She would stay with Lili, often holding her until she drifted off to sleep. Although Julie hated leaving her baby even for a few hours, the hospital staff convinced her to do so for her own sanity.

The hospital staff was wonderful and did what they could for all of their patients. Julie knew that Lili was in good hands. Occasionally, however, Julie would return to Lili's room and find her alone and crying. Seeing the fear in her baby's tears broke the young mother's heart.

As time passed, Julie felt more alone with her baby. Friends and family visited less frequently. The hospital in Ann Arbor, Michigan, was a long drive from their home in Lansing. And, while there were plenty of visitors at first, the visits decreased as time went on. Julie remembered each person and how often they visited. How she treasured her connection with a normal life of friends and family. Her mother visited often, but most of Julie's adult companionship was with the hospital staff and other mothers who had children in similar situations.

Julie had to come to grips with the loneliness. Her friends had lives of their own and living those lives meant less time to share with a troubled friend. It was her life and she was living it virtually alone.

Lili continued to improve and it became apparent that soon she would be able to go home again. This time, she would be going home to live with her family. Lili was going to get a chance at a normal life.

Although they did not know when Lili would be released, both Julie and Bruce knew they had to get ready. They had to be trained to give dialysis to keep Lili alive. It was a skill they learned quickly from the doctors.

When going-home day arrived, the staff bid a tearful farewell to their fearless Lili. Most were tears of joy that the baby they had come to love would be able to have a more normal life. But there were also tears of sadness knowing (and hoping) Lili would not have to come back. Just nine weeks old, Lili had spent eight weeks in the hospital getting to know its staff. Now she would go home and get to know her family.

Julie's home became a hospital of sorts. Everything had to be sterilized and a home dialysis machine helped cleanse Lili's blood. Visitors had to wear masks and gloves at certain times. Two nurses helped by splitting their time so one of them could be there six nights a week.

At first, Julie and Bruce relied on a nursing agency to help on the seventh day, but the help was so unreliable they gave up and covered it themselves, becoming quite adept at taking care of their Lili.

Throughout the summer, Lili continued to amaze her friends and family. The baby that was not expected to live continually beat the odds and did quite well, given the circumstances. She had surgery to repair two hernias and had numerous other treatments for health problems that surfaced. Through it all, Lili continued to prove she was in it for the long haul.

Editor's Note: When Lili was 14 months old, she was big enough and old enough to accept a kidney transplant from an adult donor. The kidney came from Julie. The young mother, who had given Lili life once, was able to do it a second time. Lili fought a tough fight and beat the odds. She has had her share of medical problems, but is doing very well, leading the life of a young child with some special needs. More than three years have passed since the successful transplant. Lili and her kidney "have a fabulous relationship," says Julie.

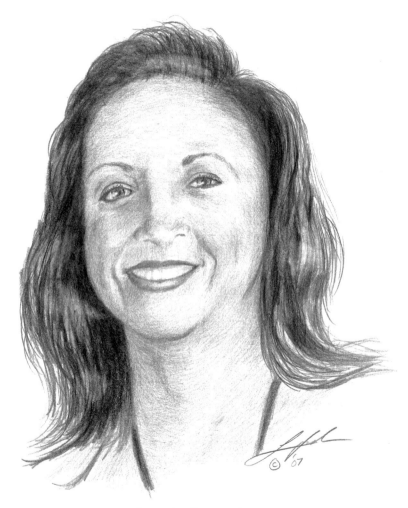

Angela Tagliaferri
Unrelated Liver Donor

20

A Gift For Mario
By Angela Tagliaferri

The Day My Life Changed Forever

I was in the passenger seat of my friend Aline's Ford Escort, taking a road trip to Pennsylvania. The windows were open and music was playing. Aline was driving, and my best friend, Francesca, was in the back seat. I don't remember what month it was, but I remember that it was a nice day.

Fran was feeling guilty for leaving her baby alone in the hospital. "I'm a bad mom. I know it...I'm a horrible mother. Do you think I'm a bad mom?" she asked. Her son, Mario, had been born a few months earlier with a liver disease called biliary artesia. He was in the hospital again, on what was one of his many hospitalizations.

"No, you're not a bad mom," I said.

What else could I say? I didn't think she was a bad mom at all. Although I'm not a mom, common sense tells me I know a good mom from a bad one. Mario was in and out of the hospital a lot, and it was taking its toll. Fran is probably the strongest person I know, but she was way beyond stressed. She went to the hospital every day and watched as her son got sicker and sicker. The doctors kept saying, "We have to wait and see," every time a question was asked.

Francesca had an 11-month-old daughter to care for, too. I had suggested she take a day off from the hospital to hang out. The change of scenery would do her good. She finally relented and agreed to take a road trip with the girls, but now the guilt was setting in.

"But I should be there. I'm his mom. What if he wakes up and I'm not there?"

Fran had been torturing herself about her son for a long time. Mario was unplanned, and raising two small children so close in age was not an idea she initially was happy about. She regretted the thought of having another child, but the regret lasted only for about 10 minutes. Those 10 minutes would haunt her for the rest of her life.

When Fran's water broke at 24 weeks, she blamed herself. When the doctor told her she had to remain in the hospital on bed rest, she dutifully laid there like it was her punishment. And when Mario was born nine weeks premature with this illness, the guilt kept piling on. Every horrible thing that happened to that child was Fran's penance for those 10 minutes of doubt.

"Well, I don't know if I told you, but the doctor says he'll definitely need a transplant someday," Fran continued.

Wow, a transplant? The only thing I knew about transplants is that people waited a really long time and sometimes died waiting. My friend Wendy's daughter had been on 'the list,' but that was about 20 years ago. It was the closest I had ever come to knowing someone in that situation.

In the car that day, I didn't make the connection that Wendy's daughter, Amber also had needed a liver transplant. (Some time later I learned that Amber suffered from the same disease as Mario. Back then, living liver donation was not an option and Amber died because no liver became available. Wendy was too afraid to ever have more children. It still surprises me that, in pictures of Amber and Mario, the two look almost identical.)

"Did you know that a liver transplant can be done with a living donor?" asked Fran. "The doctor told us as long as you're the same blood type, they can run other tests to see if you're a match. If all the tests go through, you can give away part of your liver, and it grows back!"

Grows back? Well that's the oddest thing I'd ever heard! An organ that grows back? If I hadn't been so focused on the seriousness of the situation, I would have said, "Cool!"

Fran went on, "I already know I'm blood type B because of all the tests they ran when I was pregnant, so I can't donate."

I remember not thinking too much about the statement at the time, other than feeling for Fran and trying so hard to be compassionate about something I obviously knew so little about. "You don't have the same blood type as Mario? What type does he have?"

"He's O positive."

"Huh, really? Isn't that funny.... I think I'm O positive...."

My Offer to Donate

As the months passed, Mario kept getting sicker. He could barely keep any food down. He wasn't growing, either; at five months old he was still the size of a newborn. He never seemed to catch up in size. His skin and eyes always had a yellowish tint. Sometimes he would cry for hours and could not be consoled.

About this time, I had a routine physical so I asked to have my blood typed. I wanted to see if my blood type was indeed the same as Mario's. The doctor confirmed that it was.

I called Fran later that day to let her know that I was willing to be a liver donor for Mario. "I just wanted to let you know I'm O positive. I had the doctor confirm it."

"Oh...that's so sweet of you! The doctors are pretty sure that Joe must be O positive. Since I'm B, it makes sense that Joe is O."

"Okay. I just wanted to throw it out there in case you need me."

"That's nice of you to offer. That means so much to me that you would even get your type tested! Thanks!"

We laughed about it that day. "Damn, I wanted you to be indebted to me forever," I said.

The Call

I was home alone one night when Fran called. She frequently called from the hospital after Mario fell asleep. Her voice was unusually distant and quiet, and very, very sad.

Fran explained that, unless Mario had a transplant, there was no way he would live to be two or three years old. They needed to wait a few months so he could gain some weight, but then he would need a liver transplant.

I could hear Joe crying in the background, not because his child needed a transplant, but because his blood type was incompatible and he could not be Mario's donor.

At any other time I would have cracked a joke about Mario's paternity. Fortunately I was quick enough to catch my mouth in time.

I couldn't understand how both parents could be

incompatible with their own child. It didn't make sense to me. They both had type B blood, yet their baby was O positive. I wished I had paid more attention when they taught this in school.

Before I could even begin to comprehend this whole conversation, Fran asked softly, "Remember when you told me Mario could have your liver?"

She sounded like she was about to cry and Fran never cries. That was all I needed to hear.

"You tell me when and where. I'll be there," I assured her.

Testing

The three of us sat in the room together waiting for the surgeons. Fran and Joe had told Mario's doctors that I was willing to be a donor. The first step in the process was meeting with me to make sure I wasn't crazy or getting paid off.

The surgeons seemed pleasant and asked some questions about me and my motivation to donate. They told us a little bit about the surgery, statistical outcomes and a little bit about their background and training.

I wanted to know about my health in the future, but that wasn't something they could answer. It was 2001 and transplants from living liver donors had only been an option for about 12 years. No data had been collected on donors' long-term health risks. I would have to base my decision on what little was known.

The outcome for Mario, however, seemed like a sure-fire win. "He'll be playing high school football," we were told. "He'll pull through, no problem." The possibility of Mario not surviving was never mentioned.

Because of Mario's size, only about 20 percent of my liver would need to be transplanted into him. After a few months, the missing piece of my liver would grow back. The small portion in Mario would expand to fit his abdominal area and would continue to grow as he grew.

To see if I were a suitable donor, the testing would be done in three stages: blood tests, a CAT scan and an angiogram. Once I 'passed' each stage, I could move to the next, with an opportunity to back out at each stage.

I passed the blood tests with flying colors. No diseases, no problems. Other than returning to work afterward woozy and light-headed, it was uneventful. When they mixed my blood with Mario's, there were no adverse reactions.

The same was true with the CAT scan. After looking at the size and shape of my liver, the doctors thought I was turning out to be a great candidate. It helped that I was smaller than average for an adult.

Marla, the nurse practitioner, called after the CAT scan to tell me I moved on to stage three, the angiogram. It sounded like it was no big deal.

"They'll put a tube in your leg and shoot some dye into the vein. The dye will travel up to your liver and they will be able to look at the veins and arteries of your liver, kind of like a road map. If they feel your 'mappings' match Mario's liver, that will be it for the testing."

That didn't seem too traumatic, so I wasn't worried. She continued, "You'll probably have to stay at the hospital a couple hours after the test. When they remove the tube they want to make sure the incision clots, so they'll keep you a few hours before letting you go home."

When I arrived at the hospital the next day, I was handed a gown and instructed by a male nurse to take off all of my clothes except my bra and gown.

The room was a big, bright room with what looked like an operating table in the middle. The nurse gave me an injection with a big syringe.

Within minutes, I was numb from the waist down and felt myself calm down. When the doctor made the incision I raised my head and saw his hand entirely covered in blood, almost up to the wrist. I remembered thinking I should be scared, but all I could do is lay my head back down. I closed my eyes and tried to think of anything else except what was going on around me, but I couldn't concentrate on anything else.

In recovery, a doctor asked me how I was getting home and if anyone had come with me. I was still under the effects of the anesthesia and it took me a minute or so to comprehend his question. I had come by myself and intended to drive home, and I didn't see why this was a problem.

The doctor explained that I was not allowed to drive. The leg had to remain as still as possible for the rest of the day. Driving would cause me to move my leg, which could cause the clot to open. "Do you live with someone?" he asked.

"No. I live alone."

He then instructed me not to take any pain medications as I would need my wits about me if anything should happen. I would need a clear head to call 911 because no one would be around to call for me.

I remember being angry at not having had this information beforehand, but before I had a chance to formulate that thought he pulled the tube out of my groin. I have never felt so much pain in my life.

Everything around me went white, then black. I screamed out loud and my hands flew out to grip the metal bars of the bed. Tears leaked out of my eyes even though they were squeezed shut, and I almost passed out.

"I have to put pressure on the opening to get the vein to clot," the doctor said. Before that had a chance to register, he was leaning on my groin with his full body weight. I didn't think I was going to make it. I was whimpering like a wounded animal. I was begging him to stop, but I don't remember if I said it out loud or only in my head.

Later, I was moved to a hospital room. When I took a peek under the covers, I discovered the entire right side of my body was swollen and bruised. The bruise extended from my stomach to halfway down my thigh. Apparently I didn't clot and was bleeding internally, and the doctor needed to try to clot the incision again. This was the routine for the next few hours, until the doctor was finally satisfied that I wasn't going to bleed to death.

I managed to find someone to give me a ride home.

"Remember," the doctor warned. "No pills. If you feel like something is wrong or are in a lot of pain, call me. If you can't stand the pain, call 911 immediately, "

Over the next few days, I tried to call him a few times. I didn't know if the pain I was in was 'normal' or 'too much.' The doctor never picked up the phone or responded to my pages. I was very scared and very alone.

I was in so much pain I could hardly move. The bruising and swelling were disgusting; the skin on the right side of my body from belly button to thigh was black, and every part that was bruised was also extremely swollen. I could barely walk, let alone sit or get into a car. My vagina was so swollen on the right side that when I tried to go to the bathroom, urine would spray down my left side. Every time I went to the bathroom I was crying and laughing at the same time; my predicament seemed ridiculous and crazy and scary; and no one at the hospital seemed to care.

The angiogram was on a Thursday and, on the following night, Marla called me at home to let me know I had passed all of the tests. The transplant team had determined I couldn't be a more perfect match. I was elated. It was all worth it. Although I was bruised and battered, I would be Mario's donor.

Marla encouraged me to think about it over the weekend and assured me I could change my mind and back out. They could simply tell Fran and Joe that I was not a suitable donor. My mind was already made up. I had been peeing on my leg for two days – I had done nothing but think about it. If they wanted to wait a few days, they could, but I was going to call Fran and give her the good news. I would be Mario's donor.

About two weeks later, on Halloween, Joe brought Mario to work dressed up like a pea in a pod. We walked around and I showed off how cute Mario was in his costume. He weighed only about eight or nine pounds, so no one could believe he was already seven months old. I didn't bother explaining.

Fran and Joe went off at one point to talk to some coworkers, leaving me alone with Mario sleeping in my arms. I sat down and looked at his face and felt like all the wind got knocked out of me. It was then that the enormous magnitude of what I was doing hit me; I was really going to save this person's life. He was sick, and a part of my body was going to be removed in an effort to give him the life he couldn't have on his own. I started crying as I bent down and kissed his forehead. It was then I felt our bond.

"From now on kid, we're a team."

Time Passes

We had everything prepared and ready for the transplant. Insurance matters were arranged. At work and at school, everyone was aware that things could happen quickly. Although the surgery was scheduled for December 13, we were prepared in case of emergency.

Mario kept getting sicker and sicker. He still made frequent trips to the hospital. He went back again in late November; he had developed cholangitis (an infection) and needed antibiotics.

I went to Fran's house one day while she was cleaning. She was completely on edge. Mario was obviously very, very sick and the doctors still didn't have answers. Like any infant, when Mario didn't feel well he cried constantly. Fran wasn't getting much sleep and she couldn't understand why they just wouldn't do the transplant.

"I can't stand this," she said. She was putting clothes away in the closet with such force I was surprised they weren't ripping in half.

"He's sick. He's in the hospital again. They don't even know what's wrong with him. I keep telling them they should just do the damn transplant already. I mean, what are we waiting for?! We have the donor. You're ready. He obviously needs it now, so why wait until December? But they keep fluffing me off like I don't know what I'm talking about. I mean really, I'm just his mother, what the heck would I know?"

I kept my mouth shut and just stood there. All of a sudden she stopped what she was doing and turned to face me.

"You know what I think? I think my son is going to die. I know it – I'm his mother and I can just feel it – my son is going to die. I am going to end up burying my child."

I was silent for a moment, and then I said, "I'm not doing the transplant."

"What?"

"Fran, I am risking my life for you. I'm risking my life and my health and God knows what else for your son, and you're going to stand here and tell me he's going to die? That you KNOW he is going to die? Then why am I doing this?! Why should I risk my life and my health for him if he's going to die anyway?"

I got in her face and said, "I need you to believe. I

need you to believe in me. I need you to believe that this is going to work. If you don't believe I'm doing this because it's going to save your son's life, then there's really no point, is there?"

We stood there, just staring at each other. Very quietly she said "Okay, I'll believe this will work and he's going to live."

I turned around and walked out.

To this day, Fran and I have never talked about that conversation. We have rehashed every other detail of this story, but never that day. I don't know if she even remembers that conversation. If she does, she knows better than to say, "I told you so."

December 13, 2001

The day of surgery had come at last. I was in the hospital with my Mom and Dad, and I was yelling at the receptionist, but I don't remember why. I was nervous and on edge and ready to jump out of my skin.

We took a few photographs and I wondered if Mario had any idea what was happening.

I was taken back and given a gown. I was weighed and checked over, each step being recorded on the charts. When the preliminary work was done, I went back to the pre-op where my parents and friends were waiting. There was more paperwork to fill out and another consent form to sign.

Then another doctor came in. It's then that I learned for the first time that they would be taking veins out of my leg.

"My leg? Why are you taking veins from my leg?!"

They explained something about the piece of liver they would remove not having enough "connectors" to attach it into Mario, so they needed additional veins from my leg to attach it properly. I wondered what else I hadn't been told.

The surgeons came in and said it was time. My heart started pounding and I was getting nervous. Fran gave me a hug and let me kiss Mario. I gave her my crucifix to wear. I had worn that crucifix since the day the testing began, refusing to take it off until that moment.

Joe came over, with tears in his eyes. He bent down, gave me a hug and whispered softly, "Thank you for saving my son's life."

"You're welcome," I smiled.

As they started to take me to the operating room, my mom smiled, and my dad started to cry. They put a needle in my arm and told me to start counting backward from 100. I couldn't even say "one hundred" before I fell asleep.

It seemed like only a moment later when I opened my eyes. I could barely keep them open for more than a second. I asked the nurse when the surgery would start.

But the transplant had already taken place, and I was in recovery.

I was fighting to keep my eyes open, not believing it was over. I touched my face and could feel tubes coming out of my nose.

A few hours later, I was taken to a room on the other side of the hospital. It was huge, and I had it to myself. Since Mario was a baby, we had the surgery in the children's hospital, which is where he would stay. I moved to the adult transplant floor, where I would stay with transplant recipients.

A large group was in my room that night. All of my family, Fran's family and most of Joe's family were there to see if I was okay, and some of my friends also stopped by. I was touched.

I was completely loaded on morphine to hide the pain. Most of the night I had a death grip on the rails of the bed, as I was convinced I was sliding off onto the floor. I kept falling asleep in the middle of my sentences, only to wake up five seconds later and start them again where I left off.

The doctors told us that Mario had come out of the surgery with flying colors. His old liver was nothing more than a little rock, and they were surprised he had liver function at all. I was elated to find out he was recovering. Everybody was in a joyous mood. The surgery worked and I had saved Mario's life.

A few days later, though, everything changed. Mario's liver had shut down. He was not rejecting the liver, but there wasn't enough blood flow to the liver. The problem, the doctors explained, had something to do with how the liver had been 'sewn in.' It was now failing, and Mario would need another transplant or he would die.

I was still in a morphine haze and didn't fully grasp what the doctor had told us. Did they just admit to sewing the liver in wrong? Was I hearing things? Mario might die?

Fran and Joe had talked to the doctors earlier and were frantic to find another donor. Because everyone in Fran's family had B positive blood, none of them was suitable. Joe has two siblings; one would not get tested and the other had her blood type tested when Mario first got sick. She was his blood type, but decided to not pursue the rest of the testing. She stood there with Fran and Joe as they got the news of the required transplant, but remained silent.

Fran came back to my room after visiting Mario and said she could tell something wasn't right. She told me, "That's not my son lying in that bed." I didn't know what she meant.

Mario ended up receiving a liver from a deceased donor two days later. Doctors told me my veins were used to attach the second liver, as if hearing a part of me was still in him would somehow make me feel better.

Over the next few weeks, Mario went through a battery of tests and three more surgeries. His new liver was functioning but his kidneys had shut down, so he was on constant dialysis. He had suffered brain damage but no one could (or would) tell us why.

I left the hospital a week after my surgery. The doctors wanted me to stay longer but I refused. I just wanted to go home.

Christmas Day

I spent the night at my brother's house on Christmas Eve because I wasn't allowed to drive, and I wanted to be with my nieces on Christmas morning as they opened presents.

I called Fran at the hospital and wished her a Merry Christmas.

Fran gave me the bad news: "Mario is going to die."

Tears started rolling down my cheeks. She told me the pediatric hepatologist had spoken to them in the elevator the night before and told them Mario was "almost brain dead." How could you be "almost" brain dead?

Against doctor's orders I drove to the hospital that night. Everyone yelled at me, but I didn't care. I walked up to Mario's bed and just stared at him. He was going to die. This was really happening.

It was hard see him that way. He was hard to look at. His eyes constantly rolled around and around, back into his head with only the whites visible. His hands were balled into tight fists, and his whole body shook. He always had a look on his face like he was crying, but no sound came out.

The doctor in charge told Fran and Joe to start making some decisions. They had to decide if they wanted to take him off life support. There was no telling how long he would survive; he could become very sick and die in the hospital or he could remain that way for years. If they didn't want to remove support they would have to institutionalize him. And if Mario outlived his parents, the responsibility of his care would fall on his sister, who was still a baby.

The New Year

After the New Year began, Fran, Joe and I sat down with the doctors from the Pediatric Intensive Care Unit (PICU) to discuss Mario and his care. When we finally got a straight and honest answer, we learned that Mario was in a persistent vegetative state.

We questioned whether the transplant team had Mario's best interest in mind. They treated him as a success because he had a functioning liver, but the PICU doctors were looking at the bigger picture. In the words of one of the doctors, the transplant team was doing things to him rather than for him. Mario would never have the quality of life we all wanted and expected.

The three of us recounted the story of Mario's liver and the 'problem' with how it had been 'sewn in.' Even though we were told the story separately, we each heard the same thing. But the transplant team denied ever saying that.

We learned for the first time that Mario was in liver failure during November when he was being treated for an infection. At one point, I had to hold Fran back. I was certain she was about to get up and either start screaming or hit someone. If her son was in liver failure in November, why hadn't she been told?

They said they told us, but we must not have understood.

We learned that Mario's brain damage had occurred after the first transplant but before the second. That just added to Fran's anger. "Not only did they waste your liver, they wasted someone else's liver, too," she later said.

Fran and Joe were being asked what they wanted to do about Mario, but how do you make a decision like that? How do you decide to take your son off life support? Fran decided to ask Mario.

She stood at Mario's bedside. "Mario, it's Mommy," she said. "Tell Mommy what to do. Mommy doesn't know what to do and I can't make this decision. Please don't make me make this decision on my own. Tell me what you want me to do."

Shortly after that conversation, Fran and Joe got a call at about 5:00 a. m. telling them to come to the hospital immediately; Mario had flat-lined and had to be resuscitated. I already knew of Fran's conversation with Mario, and when she called later that morning to tell me what happened she had a certain sense of peace.

"He answered me. I feel in my heart this was his way of saying 'Mommy, it's okay to let me go.'"

Mario was given a 'Do Not Resuscitate' order, and Father Scott was called in to give him last rites. Fr. Scott, a constant source of encouragement through everything, had baptized Mario and given him his first communion before the surgery. Fr. Scott also performed Mario's confirmation, when Fran and Joe confirmed him with the name Angelo.

I don't think I heard one word Fr. Scott said. I just stood there, staring and crying and praying for a last-minute miracle.

Before surgery, Fr. Scott told me that giving my liver to Mario was "something that Jesus would do." Fran and I laughed for hours over that one, but no one was laughing today.

Mario's aunt put paint on his foot and took a footprint for a quilt. The nurses made his footprints in clay too. Then we all just stood around his bed and looked at him and cried. It was time to say good-bye.

There would be no miracle.

I didn't want to leave. I remember thinking this was the last time I'd see Mario. I took some pictures of Fran and Joe holding him – they were able to hold him since he had been removed from dialysis – and then I left.

On January 14, Mario died in his mother's arms.

January 17, 2002

It was the day of Mario's funeral. I was still not feeling well physically, and my heart was heavy. Fran and Joe decided against a wake and were just having a funeral service. There would be a private service at the funeral home. I would meet them at the church.

The church was packed. Not only were all the members of our families in attendance, but there were scores of people from work, too.

The pallbearers removed the casket from the hearse and I was stunned. Mario's coffin was so tiny. It looked like an elaborately decorated shoe box.

Fran invited me to walk in the church with the family. There wasn't one dry eye. I sat in the second row, because I would be giving a reading.

I don't know how I made it through the reading. I was crying and trying hard to not let my voice crack. I prayed I wouldn't pass out while walking down the steps past the altar.

After the funeral, everyone was allowed to walk past the casket one last time. I got in line, and asked myself why I was standing in line with everyone else. A part of me died with Mario that day, and I needed time to say good-bye.

Why didn't I get more time? Why couldn't I go last? Didn't I deserve more? But I was pushed through the line; and with only a brief touch to the top of his casket, I said good-bye to Mario.

* * *

My experience with the transplant center was not a great one, but I have heard of horrible experiences donors have had after their surgeries and, in comparison, mine was not that bad. I have since transferred my care to another transplant center in my area.

Mario's death was several years ago, and I still struggle every day to find a reason why I was brought into this situation. If I wasn't meant to save someone, why did I do this? I think I am finding that reason in my involvement in the organ donation community. Since Mario's death, I have:

- Become a speaker for Life Banc, an Organ Procurement Organization in Ohio.
- Attended and spoken publicly at meetings involving organ transplantation, and
- Served on the Living Donor Committee with the United Network of Organ Sharing.

If there's one thing I would like to accomplish with my work in organ donation, it is my extreme desire to teach the medical community and donors alike that the choice to be a donor is a life-long commitment. Too often, I see both the donors and the doctors treating the donation as a "surgery" – a single, finite point in time. Living donation is not a "surgery." It is a process. Donation is a choice that can and will affect your life forever. I will always be a donor, and the struggles that go along with that, whether emotional, mental, physical or financial, will be with me for the rest of my life. There are consequences to these decisions – both good and bad – and too few prospective donors put enough thought into what comes later. Being a match shouldn't be the only thing we look at.

When I had my surgery, I could not be told what my future would look like. There weren't any data available regarding a donor's long-term health. Moving forward knowing my future was uncertain was my choice, but should not be the choice the next generation of donors should have to make. The Donor Registry, a comprehensive database of information on the long-term health of donors, is my other passion.

The transplant community has worked so hard. I see progress, but much has yet to be done. This is why I want to stay involved.

I have made a very conscious choice to not "move forward" past Mario's death and get beyond it. Instead, I have chosen a difficult path: to bring my grief with me and make it a part of my everyday life. To talk about him, share our story and make Mario very much a part of the present. It was a hard choice – a very sad choice – but his memory keeps me moving forward toward change...for others as well as myself.

Author's Note

Mario was born March 11, 2001, and passed away January 14, 2002. Because this story took place many years ago, my memory of certain events is hazy. Parts of the story may be stated out of order, and conversations may not be quoted exactly. However, as best I could, I tried to capture the subject and emotion of the conversations.

This story is told from my point of view. At times throughout the story, I state a person "felt" or "thought" a certain way. Please note this is my perception of their thoughts or feelings; and may not in reality have been what they were thinking or feeling at all. My perception is my reality, not necessarily the reality.

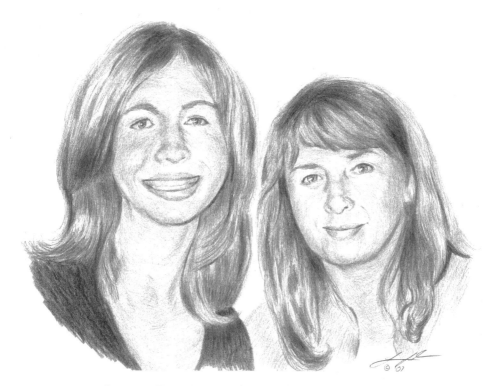

Jenna Franks
Kidney Recipient

Karol Franks
Recipient Family

21

A Test of Faith in Strangers

By Alan Zarembo

There are a billion people on the Internet, and perhaps someone, somewhere, had a kidney to spare.

"19 yr. old daughter needs O kidney," Karol Franks typed, specifying the proper blood type.

Her eldest child, Jenna, had a rare defect that destroyed her kidneys. She had been undergoing dialysis for more than a year, tethered to a machine three days a week, three hours a day, to filter toxins from her blood.

Exhausted after each session, Jenna usually retreated to her bedroom. "I'm fine," she would tell her mother before climbing the curving staircase of their spacious home.

Her daughter's youth was slipping away, Karol thought.

No friends or relatives were found to be acceptable matches for a transplant. Kidneys from cadavers are allocated primarily to those who have waited the longest, and Jenna was at least five years from the top of the regional transplant waiting list. Karol thought of getting an organ from one of her other children, but at 16, 14 and 9, they were deemed too young to donate.

With no alternatives, Karol last year turned to the Internet, though she couldn't imagine why someone would want to give a kidney to a stranger.

Money, guilt, salvation?

Karol continued typing: "Please consider donating a kidney so she can get off dialysis."

Her husband, Ed, was skeptical. He didn't place much hope in the Internet, full of scammers and kooks.

Disabled by a back injury, Ed was often resting in his room. Down the hall, Jenna was quiet in hers.

Karol remained alone downstairs at her computer.

"We are in Pasadena, CA. Thank you from a very grateful mom," she concluded and posted her message on the website http://www.livingdonorsonline.org. The return address: kidney4jenna@yahoo. com.

She said nothing about it to Jenna.

Being on dialysis is like someone hitting the "pause" button on your life, Jenna said.

She was 15 when doctors determined that her kidneys were failing, the result of pressure in her urinary system from an inability to sense when her bladder was full.

At first, Jenna refused to accept that she was sick, stashing her medicine in her dresser until the housekeeper found it and told her mother. As Jenna grew more lethargic, her defiance waned.

At the dialysis clinic, Jenna was always the youngest patient. Flopped in a padded recliner, she usually placed a pillow over her face and fell asleep.

All around her were patients who had been on dialysis for years. That was her future, she imagined.

Karol, now 52, urged her to meet other teenage kidney patients. Jenna didn't see the point.

"That is my way of dealing with it – not dealing with it," Jenna said.

Karol gave up trying to talk to her daughter about a transplant.

In an office next to the dining room, she searched the Internet for a donor, advice or just somebody to talk to.

The statistics were depressing: more than 60,000* people in the U. S. waiting for kidney transplants. The list grows by nearly 5,000 patients a year.

Fewer than 17,000 kidneys are transplanted annually. Most come from accident and stroke victims or living relatives.

About 1,500 a year come from other unrelated donors, mostly family friends.

A tiny portion – no one knows how many – come from strangers, increasingly found on the Internet.

Many doctors feel queasy about such donors. Selling organs is illegal in the United States, and they worry that patients and families will buy organs from people desperate to sell – especially from abroad – or accept them from crackpots desperate to give.

In recent years, it has become easier to find donors through websites set up for people looking for organs.

Once a deal is struck, it is not uncommon for people to pose as old friends to avoid raising suspicions from the hospital.

Karol asked herself: Was she willing to lie? Would she pay for an organ? What would she be willing to do to persuade someone to give away a kidney?

Subject: i can donate It can be some dificulties but i can

*Data as of original publication date.

donate to your daughter one of my kidneys, i'm 44 o+ good health, living in mexico

The e-mails – some in faulty English – began trickling in the day after Karol posted her plea.

Subject: We need money to cure my kid $ 30 000! I am ready to become a kidney donor.

Dear, Sir/Madam!

I will send my kidney! Kidney on sale. .. My age is 22, weight – 68 kg., height 175. Absolutely healthy. I live in Ukraine.

another.. .

Subject: POTENTIAL DONOR AVAILABLE Hi! I am 28 years old, a single mother of an 7 year old boy named Josh.... We are called Jesus Christians. We try to follow the teachings of Jesus Christ and practice these teachings in our everyday lives, which is why I am writing to you now.

Karol pondered each message, forwarding some to her husband. Ed, now 54, had a doctorate in public policy and had been a financial analyst – the family pragmatist.

He knew about hope and disappointment. In the seven years since injuring his back in a skiing accident, he had seen dozens of doctors and undergone four surgeries to relieve the constant pain. Nothing worked.

The e-mails seemed only to confirm everything he believed about the world. "I was very worried that some con man would take advantage of the situation," he said.

He responded to his wife from a laptop in bed: "No." "No way." "Wacko."

Karol knew he was probably right. But she still thought of each new e-mail as a possible kidney for Jenna.

One message stood out. It was longer than most and exuded a sincere desire to help. In fact, the sender said that he had already started testing in hopes of donating in his hometown, Salt Lake City – through a program in which the hospital chooses a recipient from its waiting list.

Subject: Possible Donor The reason I'm pursuing other possible recipients is because while my act is totally of an altruistic nature I still have the need in some small way to know that someone very deserving and most importantly very in need will receive my kidney. I am 39 years old, blood type O-and in good health.

The message, which arrived May 1, 2005, was unsigned, but Karol could see from the e-mail address that the sender's name was Steven.

She responded an hour later: "I am grateful that you wrote and I admire what you are doing." It seemed Karol was always on the Internet, searching.

Ed worried that she was becoming addicted. After years of trying to heal his back, he understood the obsession to find a cure.

But he feared his wife's quest was straining their marriage.

Karol felt alone. She began to confide in Steven, a medical courier and practicing Mormon with two children.

"I am fine most days, I have an optimistic nature, but it is just a very frustrating path and I stumble sometimes," she wrote.

Subject: Friend from Salt Lake Karol, I realize the ups and downs of this whole process for you. You will have your hopes as high as a kite one minute and down in the dumps the next. I can assure you that I will do everything I can to help your daughter.

Karol didn't know what to make of people who seemed to genuinely want nothing in return. "Are they missing something?" she wondered.

Mostly, she came to realize that everybody wanted

something, tangible or not.

One Kentucky woman was hoping to move to California with her daughter and, it turned out, was offering her kidney to anybody who could set her up with a job and a house – preferably near the beach.

Many of the messages came from people overseas seeking money.

> *Subject: kidney "30 years old male from israel in perfect health condition, blood type o+ is willing to sell a kidney. .. my availability to arrive anywhere in the world is allmost immidiatly (I have 2 passports, one of them is german-it means that i dont need any visa to most of the countries).*

Karol asked Steven what he would make of some of the e-mails offering organs for sale. It was a way of letting him know that if it was money he wanted, she wasn't interested.

> *Subject: Friend from Salt Lake I can't even imagine the frustration and disgust you must experience in reading a posting trying to negotiate the price for kidney to save your daughter. The sad truth is it is becoming more and more common. Human greed knows no boundaries and I think that is the main reason behind what I am trying to do.*

Karol offered to tell Steven anything he wanted to know about Jenna.

He wrote back: "I would never put you as a parent in the position of trying to sell me on why your daughter is more deserving than another individual."

Still, Karol worried about how to present Jenna to the world.

She set up a Web page for potential donors – http://www.xanga.com/i korn – and posted a photograph of Jenna as a toddler wearing Mickey Mouse ears. She also included a recent shot of her at a charity debutante ball.

Pretty and slight, Jenna was a bright face among the older patients advertising online.

Some of Karol's friends said Jenna appeared too happy, leading Karol to add a picture of Jenna hooked up to a dialysis machine, an empty look in her eyes.

Jenna had only an inkling of what her mother was doing – and Karol didn't tell her about Steven, who was quickly becoming her biggest hope.

Jenna hated that her mother wanted everyone to know she was sick. All the sympathy didn't bring her any closer to a kidney.

She had always been something of a loner. Now, she spent hours each day in her room playing an Internet adventure game incorporating Japanese anime. She took the character of a cute schoolgirl with a hulking sword strapped to her back.

Jenna never mentioned kidneys to her virtual friends.

Sometimes, she said, she thought about what she would do if she finally got a transplant. Maybe she would go back to school, get a driver's license, rent an apartment, even visit New York.

But she feared that a surgery could not solve all her problems. She had never done well in school. She'd never had to work or known what she wanted to do in life.

"I've just been worried that I've been using this whole kidney thing as an excuse for not doing anything with my life," she said.

After many e-mails, Karol and Steven took the next step: contacting the transplant coordinator at USC, where Jenna was on the waiting list. They knew he had the right blood type, but they needed to see if Jenna's immune system was compatible with his.

Karol had been warned that some hospitals might

turn down transplant candidates who advertised for kidneys.

She and Steven agreed to tell USC the truth about meeting on the Internet.

"I hope that we can become friends and there will be no question as to the 'how and why' of it all," Karol wrote.

"Karol, there is no need for us to be 'strangers' even though we have never met," he replied. "We are both human beings, loving parents and looking to help someone else other than ourselves. I think that makes us closer in some ways than individuals I have known my whole life."

USC eventually asked him to send his complete medical records.

He promised to do it, despite his complaints to Karol about the suspicions that hospitals had of donations from strangers.

"If I consciously and willingly make the informed decision to donate a kidney to save the life of a person I'm required to jump through hoops without end," he wrote.

Getting Steven's kidney for Jenna seemed so close now. Karol worried each time a few days would pass without a new message from him.

After one brief lapse, she dashed off an e-mail: "I am running out now – driving kids to school. Just thought of you, wondering how you are doing."

Six weeks after their first e-mail exchange, Steven sent a note saying he had to put his plans on hold for six months. His doctor in Salt Lake City, he said, wanted to monitor a mild liver condition.

Karol kept searching for donors as she began counting down six months.

She could wait if she had to. She had no choice.

Steven had been thinking about donating a kidney for a decade, ever since seeing a brochure during one of his frequent appointments to donate blood.

Over time, it became "a compulsion inside of me," he said in an interview in Salt Lake City.

He could not explain his motivation easily. It just seemed that if he had the power to help somebody, he should.

He spent months exercising – walking about five miles a day – to lose 60 pounds and resolve his liver problem, a fatty inflammation related to his metabolism. With 178 pounds on his 6-foot-4-inch frame, he thought he looked too thin in the mirror, but he hadn't felt better in years.

Finally, he got clearance to donate. He arranged for time off from work.

His wife, Nora, a school cafeteria worker, supported his decision. He told her it was something he had to do – to give his right kidney to a young woman he had never laid eyes on.

He waited for her in a hospital conference room for their first meeting. He introduced himself: Steven Paul Crump. They hugged awkwardly, and he kept thanking her for the chance to donate.

The surgery took place the next day.

The recipient was not Jenna Franks. It was a woman from Utah.

Nine days later, Steven was recovering at home when he got an e-mail from Karol. "I just thought I would write and say hello," it said.

He replied the next day: "I'm hoping that Jenna is still doing as well as can be expected."

It had been just a month since he had told Karol – falsely – that his donation plans were on hold. He knew the truth would be difficult for Karol and could not bring himself to tell her.

"I had been as honest as I needed to be," he said later in an interview. "Anything else was to spare her pain."

Four months passed before Karol found out. She had held off on contacting him, not wanting to be a bother. When she did, he finally told her.

"I hesitated in letting you know for some still unknown reason," he wrote. "Maybe I felt guilty because I wasn't able to help your daughter or maybe I thought you might think 'fantastic, Steve, but what does that do for Jenna?' I wouldn't blame you for feeling that way."

Karol felt betrayed. She pored over all their messages. There were dozens of them. Maybe she had misread them.

The e-mails seemed clear. "I am in this for the long haul," Steven had written. "No second thoughts whatsoever and if I could do it this afternoon I would."

For the first time, Karol mentioned Steven to Jenna, who didn't know what to think.

To Ed, the news seemed inevitable. "I didn't really think it was going to work out anyway," he said.

In an interview, Steven said he understood Karol's desperation but not the wrong she felt. He never promised anything, he said. He was simply paving the way to donate to somebody.

"It is my organ," he said. "I do think I have some obligation to myself that if I am going to give that gift, I have some say in who it goes to."

Jenna was just one possibility.

Steven also had been corresponding with a young man whose girlfriend in Sacramento needed a kidney.

Steven had contacted her transplant program as well.

But he made no headway with either hospital. He said he felt he was being treated as if he were doing something wrong.

He wanted USC to arrange a blood test to see if he was genetically compatible with Jenna.

Frustrated that the hospital wanted medical records first, he never sent anything.

Then, LDS Hospital in Salt Lake City, where he had originally expressed interest in donating, called to say there was a match for his kidney – a 33-year-old mother of four who had been waiting for five years.

Her immune system was highly sensitive, making her an extremely difficult match. Steven's kidney was perfect.

He was moved by her story.

Steven "is a hero not only to me but also to my children," said Wendy McDonald as her boys ran through the house in the small town of Enoch, in southern Utah, where she is finishing a degree in education.

"He thinks about other people before himself," she said. "He is very Christ like."

She has stayed in touch with Steven and his family – though she said he sometimes seems distant and reserved. When they talk, he always asks how the kidney is doing. It took months before Karol could bring herself to begin trading messages with potential donors again.

Strangely, she felt herself drawn back to Steven. She realized that she had never learned his last name or heard his voice.

But, she told him in an e-mail, she didn't want to repeat her mistakes with a new potential donor, a woman from Houston.

She and Steven hadn't corresponded in four months, but he answered the next day.

*Subject: Re: Salt Lake City Karol, there is nothing that
you said or did that made me decide to donate in Utah.
You are a well spoken and considerate human being. Your
interaction with this individual from Texas will relay the
same feelings and sincerity I was so taken by.*

Karol switched transplant programs – Scripps
Green Hospital in La Jolla seemed more receptive to
Internet matches.

The woman from Houston, a devout Christian, flew
out to undergo final tests. Jenna refused to meet with
her, saying she'd wait until the donation was certain.

When the woman turned out to have a rare kidney
defect, Jenna wondered if she had jinxed the deal:
"Maybe God was saying, 'If you're not even interested
in meeting her why should you get her kidney?'"

In September, Karol began corresponding with
Patrice Smith, a 44-year-old secretary from Wooster,
Ohio, who said she was inspired to donate after reading
an article in her local newspaper about a man who
needed a kidney.

She was scheduled to donate to him, but it turned
out that their immune systems were incompatible.

Patrice figured she could help somebody else.

She was a mother of four, a marathon runner and
long-distance swimmer. In some ways, she said, donating a kidney might simply be another test of her physical and mental strength.

Mail-in blood tests showed she was a match.

But the transplant team wanted to meet her to quell
any skepticism that she was being coerced and to make
sure she understood the risks.

Jenna and Karol met Patrice last month in the
lobby of the Radisson Hotel in La Jolla.

Jenna worried that it would be an audition, that she
would say the wrong thing. But at dinner, Patrice's

easy manner erased her fear.

"I feel like this is actually happening – this transplant thing," 21-year-old Jenna said after dinner. "I've been worried about getting my hopes up."

Ed had come around too: "If [Karol] had listened to everything I said, we probably would not have made contact with Patrice."

The transplant is scheduled for Jan. 16. Karol posted the good news on the website.

But she still checks her e-mail, just in case. There have been more than 75 messages from more than a dozen countries since she first posted her appeal.

They keep arriving.

Subject: hi! HI! My name is mario! i am 23 years old! i am in very good health! I am O+! i lost my mother 4 months ago! i really wanna help you! All i ask in return is to have a familly again!

By Alan Zarembo, Los Angeles Times Staff Writer
(First published in the Los Angeles Times, Dec. 30, 2006)
Reprinted by permission

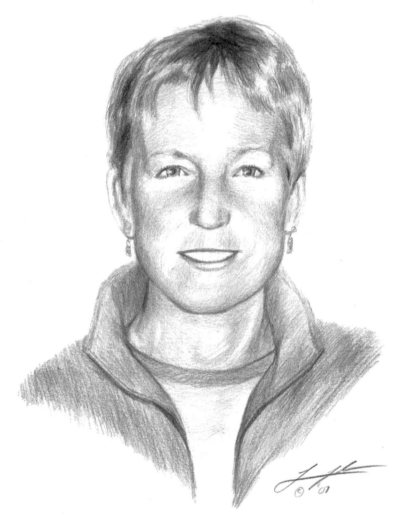

Patrice Smith
Unrelated Kidney Donor

22

Losing a Kidney, Gaining Family
By June Chandler-White

Patrice Smith is the kind of person who would give her left kidney to help a stranger. Everyone who knows her is not surprised she did.

"I wasn't surprised at all, not with her. Patrice is one of a kind, and such a compassionate person. She just felt this need to be able to help somebody because she could," said Pam Tegtmeier, recalling her reaction when she learned her best friend of 20 years planned to pay her own way to fly to California to donate an organ to a young woman she'd never met before.

It doesn't take two decades to see Smith, a secretary at The College of Wooster, mother of four, competitive swimmer and veteran marathoner, has a truly giving spirit. All it takes is her story.

It began when Smith read in The Daily Record early last year about a local man who was coping with kidney failure, dealing with dialysis, feeling his life was in limbo as he waited for a transplant. She didn't know the man in the story.

"But I just couldn't let it go," Smith recalled.

She clipped out the story and showed it to her husband, Jeff.

"I gave the article to my husband and had him read it. He said, 'You want to donate, don't you?'" Patrice Smith recalled, noting her husband was concerned for her welfare, but supported her fully, in part, Patrice joked, because after 12 years of marriage, he knows her very well.

"He said, 'Does it really matter what I think?'" Patrice Smith recalled, adding serious discussion with the entire family led to everyone agreeing donating was the right thing for Patrice to do.

With the support of her family, stepdaughters Ceason, 27, and Jordan, 25, and sons Brian, 20, and Kevin, 18, Smith's research began. In March she contacted the local kidney foundation, who put her in touch with a transplant coordinator at the University of Pittsburgh Hospital. Preliminary tests determined Smith, of Wooster, was a match for David Sherrill, the man she had read about in the paper.

"We weren't friends to start, but through the course of it, we became very close friends," Smith said, noting both hoped the transplant would take place in summer. When more tests on Sherrill determined he needed heart bypass surgery, the transplant was rescheduled for October.

Then came "awful" news. A blood transfusion during Sherrill's bypass surgery had changed the antibodies in his blood, making him incompatible with Smith for a kidney transplant.

"Three days before the transplant was supposed to take place, we had a final cross-match, and his antibody levels were high. It was awful, it was really awful," Smith recalled. "They said, 'We can't do this.'"

Smith felt devastated for her new friend, who is still waiting for a transplant. She also was confused about what had happened. Unable to answer her questions, the transplant coordinator referred Smith to an online site for donors.

"I put my questions online, and this person, Karol, answered. I was really thankful. She was very articulate and explained to me what had happened," Smith recalled.

In clicking around the Web site a little more, Smith found the story of a young woman named Jenna Franks who lived in California and needed a kidney. She sent an e-mail, and learned Jenna was the daughter of Karol, the woman who had answered her questions.

"(Karol) never told me anything about Jenna. I found her on my own, basically," Smith recalled. "I wrote to Karol (again) after I read Jenna's story. I said, 'I am the same blood type, I may be able to help your daughter.' We were both being very reserved and cautious," Smith recalled, explaining the communication was a leap of faith for all parties involved.

"She gave me the name of the coordinator of the Scripps Hospital in La Jolla. I contacted them, and I actually filled out an application," Smith said.

Within days, the transplant coordinator at Scripps contacted Smith, asking if she could arrange for her records to be sent from Pittsburgh. In November, Smith and her family were on a plane to California.

"They are very cautious out at Scripps. They required us to meet. They wanted to make sure that everything was ethical, that I was not getting paid or being coerced. I met with the social worker and the nephrologist and the surgeon, and it was the same questions, over and over; they were very thorough," Smith recalled.

She also met the Franks family – Karol and Jenna, dad Ed, James, 18, Becca, 16, and Johnny, 9.

"It was very emotional. It is hard to explain what it felt like to meet them," she said, noting because Jenna is so close to her eldest son's age, she felt a special desire to help her.

"Jenna is shy, she is incredibly confident. She is, other than this illness, a typical 21-year-old young lady," Smith said, noting she believed the media attention Jenna's story drew was overwhelming to her. For that reason, Smith said, when the surgery was scheduled for Jan. 16, Smith entered the hospital anonymously.

"The hospital said they had gotten some calls (from media) wanting to follow the story," Smith said. "I was afraid that something would happen, and I didn't want to make anyone uncomfortable."

Smith said she slept well the night before the surgery, despite having to get up to use the bathroom as medications to clear out her system did their job.

"I didn't have to drink 'the stuff,'" she said, referring to high-powered laxatives she'd heard "horror stories" about.

After 3 1/2 hours of surgery, Smith woke in the recovery room, her left kidney already busy at work in its new body. Smith admits her mind was relieved, but her stomach was upset from the general anesthesia.

"I was throwing up, and of course a new incision, it feels like you are just going to bust out," Smith, who also is a veteran of two Caesareans, recalled. "Thank God Jeff was there, because he took care of me. He did a great job."

After two days in the hospital, and the 10 outpatient days required by the hospital, Smith and her family were on the plane for home. Jan. 29, she returned to work. And less than two weeks after the surgery, she was back to doing what she loves best of all.

"I started running less than two weeks after the surgery. I am training for the Boston Marathon with Pam (Tegtmeier)," said Smith.

Just as no one who knows Smith was surprised to learn she was donating a kidney, no one was surprised to learn she was back to training for her next marathon less than two weeks later.

"We did an 18-miler the day before she left for the surgery," Tegtmeier said.

Smith acknowledges being so fit has played a large role in her quick recovery. She credits her friends and family for supporting her decision to donate.

"The closer I got, I'll admit the more scared I got, but the closer I got, the more support I got," she said. "This sounds so corny, but it did feel like it was a football team and we were at the Superbowl, I had so much support. I was just the quarterback throwing it to the receiver. It couldn't have gone any better."

There also have been some laughs.

"Did she tell you about the chocolate?" asked Smith's co-worker Kim Tritt. Smith is a known chocolate lover, Tritt said. Jenna Franks never was – until she got Smith's kidney.

"We joke around that Patrice's cravings have been transplanted," Tritt said with a laugh.

Tritt added she and her co-workers also joke Patrice had an ulterior motive in donating to a woman in California.

"A part of her always wanted to live in the warm

weather," Tritt joked.

Smith takes the joking in stride. After all, that's what friends are for, and she says she never realized until now how many she had. She also said she didn't know how much she would gain by losing a kidney.

"(The Franks) family, they are so cute, they are funny, and just very normal, and close, you can tell they are close," she said, noting she maintains regular contact with the Franks family, who calls Smith "their hero."

For the first time since her kidneys failed six years ago, Jenna Franks is able to dream of a bright future, which she hopes includes finishing college and starting a career, possibly as an actress. For Smith, that is the greatest reward of all.

"She is doing really, really good," Smith said with a big smile.

Written by June Chandler-White
(First published in The Daily Record, Feb. 12, 2007)
Reprinted by Permission

Editor's Note: Patrice Smith ran the Boston Marathon three months after her kidney donation. She completed the 26.2 mile race in 3 hours, 40 minutes, 34 seconds.

Web-Sites
There are many resources available to learn more about organ and tissue donation. Following is an alphabetical listing of web-sites believed to provide accurate and reliable information on transplantation.

Living Donors Online
www.livingdonorsonline.org Mission: We seek to be the preeminent online community for living donors, potential donors, their families and medical professionals. "Living donors" are living individuals who have given a kidney, liver, lung, bone marrow, or other organ or tissue for transplantation to another person – often a relative – in need.

National Kidney Foundation   www.kidney.org
Who We Are: The National Kidney Foundation, Inc., a major voluntary health organization, seeks to prevent kidney and urinary tract diseases, improve the health and well-being of individuals and families affected by these diseases, and increase the availability of all organs for transplantation.

OrganDonor.Gov   www.organdonor.gov
The official U. S. Government web site for organ and tissue donation and transplantation, www.organdonor.gov, is maintained by the Health Resources and Services Administration (HRSA), Healthcare Systems Bureau (HSB), Division of Transplantation, an agency of the U. S. Department of Health and Human Services.

United Network of Organ Sharing
www.unos.org   www.transplantliving.org
Our mission is to advance organ availability and transplantation by uniting and supporting our communities for the benefit of patients through education, technology and policy development.

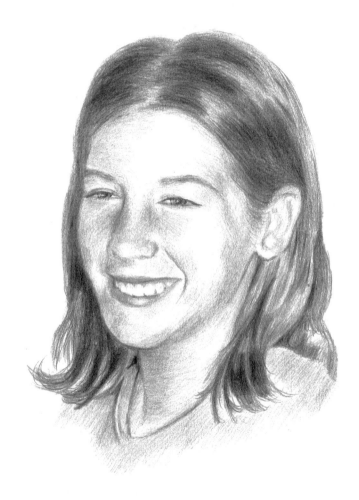

Dena McMillin
Organ, Tissue, and Cornea Donor

23

Why Wouldn't She?
She didn't need them anymore

It was the day before Dena McMillin's sixteenth birthday and her parents, Larry and Jennifer, planned a surprise birthday party. Dena was quite an athlete and many of her basketball teammates were invited. Relatives from out of town would be joining Dena in this milestone celebration. She left home with a friend to "go to dinner" so the family could decorate the clubhouse. The party was to take place in two hours and there was a lot to do. This would be a day to remember for their sweet sixteen-year-old daughter.

A telephone call interrupted the party preparation. What was intended as a surprise for Dena quickly turned into an unimaginable tragedy for her friends and family. Dena and her friend had been in an accident. The news was not good; Dena had been very badly injured. She was alive, but there was only a ten-percent chance she would live. Her friend, unfamiliar with the new neighborhood, had made a mistake.

The limbs from an overgrown tree partially covered a stop sign. In the excitement of the moment, Dena's classmate ran the stop sign she did not see. The two headed through the blind intersection across a busy two-lane highway. A Chevy Blazer struck the white sedan on the passenger side, next to Dena.

A split second earlier or later and nothing would have happened, but luck was not on anyone's side. The Blazer struck the girl's vehicle and then rolled several times. Both the father and son were thrown out of the vehicle – neither was wearing a seat belt. The mother remained inside the Blazer. Fortunately none of the Blazer's occupants were badly hurt.

The car Dena was riding in crashed into an earthen embankment coming to rest on its side. Dena was unconscious, her friend badly shaken but not injured. Only Dena would pay the price for this tragic mistake. The paramedics arrived quickly and did what they could, but there was little they could do for her. They transported Dena to Liberty Hospital, where the staff notified Dena's family to come to the hospital.

Larry and Jennifer rushed to the hospital to be by their daughter's side. Jennifer's husband Jerry was already there and had learned from the doctors that Dena's situation was very grave. The drama unfolding before them was something they could never have imagined, yet they were living it. The unimaginable drama continued to unfold before them, with parents facing realities for which no preparation is possible. It simply defied anything they ever imagined could occur to their young daughter. They wanted desperately to protect their child, and would do anything they could. But there was nothing they could do but wait helplessly as the medical professionals struggled to save Dena.

It soon became apparent that Dena would not survive. She might make it through the night, to her sixteenth birthday, but there would be no celebration.

The worst fears of the parents were suddenly becoming true. Dena stopped being Dena soon after impact. Whether she survived or not, she would never be the same. The brain was damaged, and her young life would soon end.

The tragedy of what happened to this young teenager with a bright future ahead could have been worse were it not for a chance conversation she'd shared with her mother a month before the accident. Dena had worked as a volunteer at a hospital in Kansas City, and the subject of organ donation came up. Jennifer asked her if she would be willing to donate her organs if something unexpected were to happen.

Dena's answer was short and direct. "Why wouldn't I? I wouldn't need them anymore." Although this casual conversation meant little at the time, it would be of great comfort now as Dena drew her last breaths with the help of medical machinery. At least her family knew how she felt about organ donation if she were not to survive. They could not give life back to Dena, but they could allow Dena to give life to others.

Dena died on her birthday. A day that should have been filled with anticipation of the future was instead filled with the sense of the loss from a life cut short.

When Larry and Jennifer were asked about donating Dena's organs, there was no hesitation. Their daughter had shared her views in a casual but fateful conversation with her mother. Would they donate her organs? Yes! Jennifer was comforted by remembering Dena's quick response to that fateful question a short month before.

A memorial service attended by 300 friends, family members, and fellow students was held on Sunday night. Individuals spoke about the impact that Dena had on the basketball team, the track team, and the classroom. But no one could speak of the hole left in their lives, a hole once filled by Dena.

Larry gave the last words at the service, expressing his pride in his daughter and what she was able to do in the last moments of her life. The last 36 hours had been excruciating, but some would benefit from this tragedy. Dena had become an organ and tissue donor, and she changed the lives of many people in the process.

Jennifer and Jerry remained with their darling Dena until time to remove her organs. As she watched her beautiful daughter, Jennifer thought of all the promise lost. Dena was a straight A student, talented athlete, strong and faithful Christian and such a joy. She was wonderful with children, and they seemed to idolize her. Jennifer thought of Dena's brother, David, and how he would miss his cherished little sister. They were like typical siblings growing up with scraps and arguments, but they had become very close the past year as they attended high school together. It seemed ironic that Dena had taken such good care of her body to have it end so young. Now Dena was leaving us, but her strong, healthy organs, tissue and corneas would restore quality of life to so many.

Barbera Jones of Springfield Missouri was struggling to make ends meet. She was diagnosed with emphysema in 1985 when she was three months pregnant. As the emphysema progressed, her lung capacity declined. She gave birth to a daughter, Paula, who was her pride and joy. Paula was a healthy, happy child who did not inherit her mother's disease. Things were a little tougher on mother and daughter due to the disease.

Paula had to learn to walk at a young age; her mother did not have the strength to pick her up or carry her.

Paula could only hold on to her Mother's outstretched fingers as the two struggled to walk together. The daughter struggled learning how to walk while the mother struggled with the strength to walk.

By 1998, Barbera's lung capacity had dropped to about 12 percent of normal. The decline in lung capacity was increasing and the doctor's were doubtful that she would live to the end of the year. Barbera was in desperate need of a lung transplant. Without the transplant, Barbera would certainly die.

By then Paula had become a teenager. She needed her mom but was facing the reality that she might lose her. Paula was not ready to give up her mother. Similarly, Barbera was not ready to leave her daughter. As was true for the past several years, each needed the other and was not willing to let go. They needed a miracle. The miracle came in the form of Dena McMillin's tragic death and her decision to become an organ donor.

Dena McMillin's 16-year old lungs were transplanted into Barbera Jones. This gift from Dena gave new hope for Barbera and her daughter Paula. The transplant was successful and the lungs worked. The emphysema had passed and Barbera had a renewed opportunity for life. Barbera's condition began to improve immediately and she became able to live a more normal life.

Barbera did not know where her lungs came from. She only knew they came from a teenager who was killed in an accident. Barbera would never have the opportunity to meet the girl who renewed her life, but she would be forever in her debt. Every breath she takes is in thanks to Dena's generosity.

Barbera could only wonder what Dena was like, and what it was like for her family to lose a child so young, a child with such a bright future cut short tragically. Barbera exchanged letters with the McMillins even though they did not know each other, not even each other's names. The letters were funneled through the Midwest Transplant Network so the families can correspond and still maintain anonymity. After two years of correspondence, the families decided to meet.

The meeting was arranged by a local television affiliate in Springfield, Missouri. Although it was the first time the families had met, it was as if they had known each other a lifetime. The bond they shared was stronger than familial ties. The lungs that allowed Barbera to breathe had come from this family and from their generosity.

Jennifer noticed immediately the sparkle in Barbera's eyes. "Dena had such a sparkle in her big brown eyes, and you have it too," said Dena's mom, as she tearfully embraced the recipient of Dena's lungs. "I feel so rewarded to see that Dena lives on in you."

Barbera and Paula Jones, a mother and daughter pair, are likely together today because Dena and her mother can no longer be together. Dena's death allowed Barbera to live. Miracles can happen even in times of tragedy.

Dialysis is a miracle of modern medicine which allows a person to live even when their kidneys are not functioning. It is a very uncomfortable procedure, often causing the patient to feel as though they have the flu. As Alice Walleck, a dialysis patient described it, "I always felt like I was on a leash."

For three years the 54-year-old grandmother went through the procedure. She had to do it three times a week. Each time she would spend three and a half hours hooked up to her dialysis machine. At first she had to do dialysis in the hospital. Eventually, she was allowed to do it in her home in Overland Park, Kansas.

With two large needles in her arm, the machine drew her blood from her body, ran it through a series of filters to clean out the waste, and returned it back to her. It was a procedure she would usually undergo late in the evening so she could go straight to bed afterward. The dialysis left her drained both physically and emotionally.

The process was very uncomfortable and Alice hated it. She even considered quitting the dialysis even though that would end her life. While hooked up to the machine, she would try to keep busy. She tried crossword puzzles, but that did not work. The process was too uncomfortable for her to sit up in a chair.

The need for Alice Walleck to take dialysis ended when she received Dena McMillin's kidney. Jennifer and Jerry knew Alice through their neighbor, Rita. Alice is Rita's sister and Dena was very close to Rita. Dena was aware of Alice's situation and felt Rita's concern. They knew Alice was on the waiting list for a kidney transplant, and they wanted to determine if Dena's kidney would be a match. It was.

Alice had just returned from the casino that Sunday evening when she got the call. She'd won $150 and considered it her lucky night, but the prize she took home from the casino paled in comparison to the gift she would receive from the sixteen-year-old Dena.

It is rare for an organ recipient to meet her deceased donor. But these were special circumstances because this was to be a direct donation. Jennifer really wanted the kidney to go to Alice because she knew Dena would want that.

Alice met the family at Liberty Hospital. Alice was allowed to see Dena for the first time as she lay in a hospital bed. Dena's family was with her as her final moments of life passed.

"It was a very emotional time," said Alice, "How can you thank someone for what they are doing?" As she sat next to Dena, Alice took the young girl's hand and kissed it. She thanked Dena for what she was about to do and then left.

Soon after Dena died, her kidney was transplanted into Alice Walleck. The kidney worked well for Alice and allowed her to be freed from the dreaded dialysis machine. Her color returned to normal and so did her life. Although she has to take a large quantity of pills each day, she considers that a very small price to pay.

For a variety of reasons, the organ bank requests that donors and recipients not communicate directly for at least a year after the transplant. The two families honored this request and communicated only through Alice's sister Rita. The McMillin family draws great comfort in knowing Dena's kidney allowed Alice to return to good health. Dena lives on through a generous gift to the sister of a family friend.

* * *

Losing a child is an unimaginably tragic experience. The tragedy is compounded when the child is so young and so loved. But for the McMillins, the tragedy was softened somewhat because of the tremendous gifts their daughter gave others.

Dena had made the decision to donate her organs, and had made her decision known to her family. The family honored her decision while facing events they could never have imagined. In the end, Dena gave the gift of life to so many people.

Dena's lungs were donated to Barbera Jones allowing her life to continue.

Dena's kidney was donated to Alice Walleck to free her from a life of dialysis, a procedure that greatly compromised her quality of life.

A 36-year-old mother who was in a coma received Dena's liver. She awoke from her coma and can now sit in bed and hold her children.

A 42-year-old man has Dena's heart.

In all, more than 75 people benefited by Dena's generosity. Dena donated her organs and tissues to others. After all, why wouldn't she? She did not need them anymore.

Dena's Legacy

A woman with three young children had already received a transplant of a much-needed organ. Her liver had failed, but now Dena's gave her new life.

Another woman had been scheduled to receive a kidney transplanted from Dena. This would dramatically change her life allowing her to be freed from the dialysis that kept her alive. She had been near death, but had been given a second chance.

Other organs and tissue were used to aid those in need. Some seventy-five people in all benefited from Dena's passing. Only one would ever meet Dena, but all would be forever in her debt. She was generous to the end giving up precious gifts. Why wouldn't she? After all, she did not need them anymore.

Dena should have been opening birthday presents that day, but she did not need them. Instead of opening gifts for herself, she would be giving gifts to others.

By donating her young organs to others, Dena could live on. The loss that the McMillin family experienced on that June day would allow others to experience a better life. Dena's parents would give anything to have their daughter back again, but it was not meant to be. They would have to settle with the knowledge that Dena's organ donation would allow her to live on in others.

Dena's father draws comfort in knowing she was able to help others after her death. "This proves the organ donation program works," said Larry. This proud father lost his only daughter and would give the world to get her back. Faith allowed him to say good-bye knowing that Dena was headed to everlasting Heaven.

Drawing what little comfort he could from this situation, Larry said, "You shouldn't feel about the loss. You should feel about the gain. I feel so rewarded that Dena lives on in others."

* * *

Donor Dad deals with the loss of a teenager

The feeling of loss never goes away. But as a Donor Dad, there are differing ways of dealing with the loss of a loved one. In my case, seeing what a life changing difference donations can make in the life of another, gives me comfort in knowing we made the right decision to donate my 16-year-old daughter's organs and tissues.

I decided that becoming involved in organ and tissue donation awareness programs was a way to continue to honor my daughter and give hope to others. Stressing the importance of having a family discussion and knowing what your loved one would want to do is the most important goal of the awareness program. It's not easy speaking in front of 300 high schools students about why we made the choice to donate. Even harder to look into the eyes of those young teenage girls and think, that if I had just held Dena for 30 seconds more, then the accident would never have occurred. But my strong faith makes me trust the Lord that Dena's death was part of his plan for all of us.

So my gift to each donor family is to encourage you to look into possibilities to mentor other donor families. Look for ways to become involved, by telling others the message of a second chance at life. If you lose a loved one, make sure some good comes out of it for another.

By Larry McMillin, Dena McMillin's Father

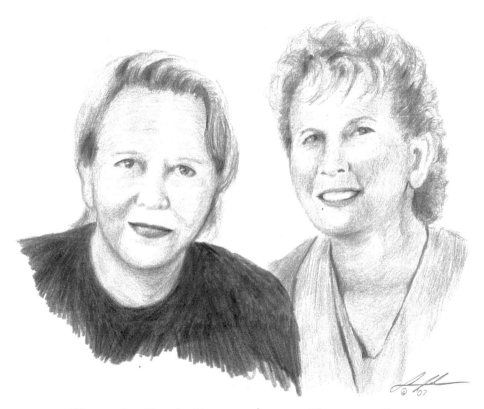

Slavenka Drakulic
Kidney Recipient

Christine Swenson
Kidney Donor

24

Meeting My 'Angel'

By Slavenka Drakulic

There she was, entering the room at the hospital in Providence, Rhode Island, in a wheelchair pushed by a nurse. For days now I had been consumed by curiosity about her. I wanted to see what kind of person possessed such generosity. Ever since I had been told that I was having the transplant surgery, I had tried to imagine her face. When I arrived on the day of the operation, I wondered: would I recognize her? Would she look special? I wanted to meet her, but would she want to meet me? She had no obligations towards me; she could have said no. Why should she meet me? She wanted to help someone who needed a kidney, not me in particular.

Now I was finally seeing her in front of me, a good-looking young woman with a fine-boned pale face, intense green eyes and short blonde hair. She was dressed in a plain grey sweatshirt and blue sweatpants. Slightly bent to the left, she kept her hand on the incision. Even though she was sitting down I could tell that she was tall and slim. Here comes my own "angel", I thought.

"Christine Swenson," she said simply, shaking my hand firmly. She looked at me. The room was full of people – her mother, her stepfather, a nurse – but in that moment I saw only her. Facing Christine was the strangest experience in my life. I do not know who smiled first, maybe we smiled at the same time. A delicate, joyful moment when we realized we were no longer strangers, that we liked each other.

For an awkward moment we were all silent. Absurd thoughts were running through my head about how I looked to them and if they would like me. I desperately wanted all three of them to feel good about the person who got her gift. I must have been a frightful sight: my hair was greasy, my face swollen from medicine, and there were tubes sticking out of my body. The room smelt of disinfectant, sweat and medicines – hardly a fitting stage for a miracle of new life.

I was overwhelmed with feelings of gratitude towards Christine, but also of tenderness. Incapable of finding any other appropriate words for her, I just said: "Thank you, thank you for saving my life." Christine looked at me, and I saw that she blushed. She must have thought I was being too theatrical. She might have improved my life, but saving it?

I knew nothing about Christine, nor did she know anything about me. Quickly, almost breathlessly, as if this would be my only chance to win her over, I told her about my 25 years struggling to survive on haemodialysis, before my first transplant, then again on dialysis. I guess I wanted to prove to her somehow that I deserved her kidney, that I had suffered enough all these years. It was as if she had been the judge who decided it was to be me.

I wanted to know so much about Christine, about her family – she told me she had a husband and two children

– and how she had decided to become a donor. Above all, I wanted to know why she had made the decision.

The story of my second transplant really begins on 11 July 2004. On that day the local newspaper, The Providence Sunday Journal, published a long report about a 21-year-old altruistic donor called Kristy Olivet. She wanted to donate her kidney and went to the Rhode Island Hospital because she had heard that its transplant surgery department had such a program.

Her kidney, doctors decided, fitted a 65-year-old man, Albert Raposa. After reading that report in the paper, five women and two men volunteered to donate their kidneys in the same hospital. I was amazed that one single story could have had such an effect. For a moment I was even proud of being a journalist, in spite of the cynicism we journalists often develop.

Christine was one of these five women. When she read the article she thought: "I could save someone's life." "Just like that?" I asked her, still incredulous, even though her kidney was already in my body. She was silent for a moment. Her answer was disarming: "Yes, just like that," she said, as if there was no need for an explanation of such an act.

But I needed to understand why she did it, because for me the comprehension of her act was a part of accepting her gift.

I asked her again the next time we met. She had invited me to her house in a suburb of Providence. We sat in the dining room, not yet friends because we knew so little of each other, but there we were face to face, donor and recipient. That's who I was to her, a recipient of her kidney. As I sat there, I touched my belly. I did not feel the kidney itself, just the incision, still fresh but no longer painful. Ten days had passed since the surgery. It was a very strange feeling to sit opposite a person, a part of whom is in you. Was it her kidney? Or was it mine now?

Christine's children, Sean, 11, and Tori, eight, were at school, her husband was at work. "Did you tell them about the surgery? Were they afraid?" I asked her. "My kids are my life. I would never do something that would leave them without a mother," she said. "I told them: 'Your mom is healthy. I am helping someone who lives with the help of a machine.'"

"I saw that they were a bit worried, but in their school classes they said they were proud of me. Tori said, just the other day, that she, too, would like to donate a kidney when she turns 18!"

Then I asked her: "Christine, what if one of your kids should one day need a kidney?"

"I would hope somebody would come forward to help, as I did," Christine said. She said it as if nothing could shake her confidence in human beings. Christine was teaching me optimism: without using these words, she taught me that people are good, that I should never doubt it.

"But how about yourself? Were you afraid of the surgery?" She brushed off the suggestion with a wave of her hand. "No, no, I did not even consider any complications. I am very healthy. No. I was not afraid."

Talking to friends back home, I realized that to them the news about my altruistic donor was no less amazing. They, too, demanded an explanation. Why did Christine do it? Is she perhaps religious? Did she do it for money? As if altruism itself is not comprehensible enough, not so self-evident a motivation. No doubt there is something shocking about a stranger giving you her kidney as a gift, because this is not what strangers normally do.

When I first saw her, I thought of her as an "angel". There, in Christine's home, I was getting angry with myself for succumbing to a cliché. She was not an angel. The beauty of her act lay in the fact that she was a perfectly ordinary person capable of such sublime altruism, kindness, generosity, largesse, goodness and excellence. It is difficult to give a name to what she has done; how much easier it is to name and describe the other, darker side of the human soul.

By labeling such people as extraordinary, we mean that we, the ordinary ones, would not be able to be either that generous or that monstrous. This might be our way of dealing with the banality of evil, but also with the banality of good. Goodness belittles you – I felt it so strongly when Christine came to my room as an ordinary person, and a stranger at that, who had committed an act of altruism.

It makes you insecure. You are not sure if you would be capable of the same thing, and you hate yourself. You see yourself as selfish, egocentric – and that is acceptable but only as long as you believe it is how normal people are. But human beings can be good and evil – not what we expect to learn about ourselves.

Again I touched my incision. Her kidney was inside me, and I could not but ask myself: what are we, Christine and I, to each other now? Are we related in some strange way? Has the kidney transplant turned us into something close to relatives? With her kidney in me, I am flesh of her flesh. We are relatives, although nobody knows what kind. And Christine didn't seem confused about how to define our relationship. "I gave a kidney and gained a sister," she stated later.

I, however, got more than a kidney and a younger sister. I got faith in ordinary goodness. I got a chance to be good to others. Because of Christine I got into a situation where I could focus less on my own needs and my worries – and that is a big gain.

By Slavenka Drakulic
(First published in The Independent, May 23, 2006)
Reprinted by permission

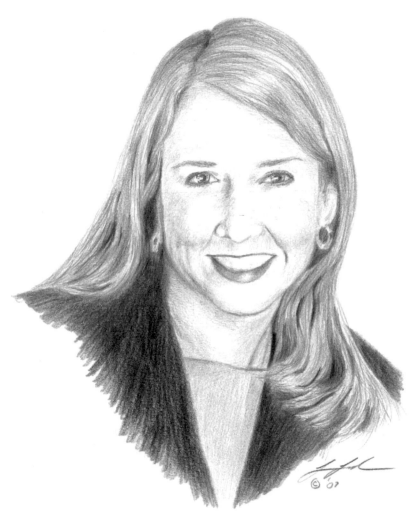

Virginia Postrel
Unrelated Kidney Donor

Here's Looking at You, Kidney
How and why I became an organ donor — and how I kept people from talking me out of it.

By Virginia Postrel

Until last November, I'd never thought about being a kidney donor. I hadn't known anyone with kidney disease, and like most people, I hadn't filled out an organ donation form when I'd gotten my driver's license. I'd never even donated blood. That all changed after I ran into a friend and asked, "How's Sally?" I got an unexpected answer: "She's... all right," in a tone that made it clear she was most definitely *not* all right.

Sally Satel and I have been friends since 1997. We're kindred spirits – strong-willed, intellectual iconoclasts who are a bit too ingenuous for our own good. But she lives in Washington, D. C., where she's a fellow at a think tank, and I live in Dallas. We almost never see each other and communicate mostly by e-mail. We follow each other's work but don't share our day-to-day lives. Last fall, no one would have called us close.

So I had no idea Sally's kidneys were failing. She needed a transplant, our friend told me. Otherwise, she'd soon be on dialysis, tied at least three days a week to a machine that would filter poisons from her blood. For someone who prizes her independence and freedom of movement as much as Sally does, dialysis would have been a prison sentence.

With no spouse, children, siblings, or parents to offer her a kidney, I thought she must be desperate. I knew the chances of getting a cadaver kidney were low, although I didn't realize how truly miniscule: More than 66,000* Americans are on the waiting list for the 6,700 or so cadaver kidneys that are available each year. Just thinking about her situation made my heart race with empathetic panic.

"Maybe we can do something to get Sally a kidney," I said. It probably sounded as if I were proposing a publicity campaign. After all, she and I and our mutual friend are in the persuasion business: We write books and articles and have lots of press connections. What I really meant, though, was "Maybe I can give Sally a kidney." At the time, it seemed like a perfectly natural reaction.

Usually when someone is seriously ill, all you can do is lend moral support and maybe cook some meals or run a few errands. Nothing you do will make that person well. But if you donate a kidney, you can (with the help of a team of medical specialists) cure her. Who wouldn't want to do it? I had no idea what a strange thought that was.

*Data as of original publication date.

Nor did I sort through my motivations. I've spent a good bit of my life trying to save the world, mostly by working to beat back bad government policies, including some that would have stifled medical research. But even when your side wins, the victory is incremental and rarely permanent. And people of goodwill dedicated to the same good cause can be awfully contentious about how to achieve their goals.

In this case, there was something reassuring about the idea that the benefit wouldn't depend at all on my talents, persuasiveness, or intellect. It would be simple. All I had to do was show up. In middle age, I've realized that I can't save the world. But maybe I could save Sally. Someone had to.

Except for living in Texas, I was the ideal candidate. I was healthy, with no family history of kidney disease. Like Sally, I had no kids depending on me. (Unlike her, I had a big family of potential kidney donors, just in case.) I was self-employed, and my husband, a professor, had a fairly flexible schedule. Neither home nor work obligations would pose a problem.

But first I had research to do. I didn't want anyone to know I was considering the idea unless I was absolutely sure I'd go through with it. I didn't want to get Sally's hopes up and then renege. That would have been worse than not volunteering in the first place.

An hour on the Internet told me what I needed to know. All a donor and a recipient have to have in common is a compatible blood type; anti-rejection drugs take care of the rest. For the donor, the operation isn't especially risky or particularly difficult to recover from. Laparoscopic techniques have replaced the old sidesplitting gashes with a few tiny holes and an incision two- to three-inches long, just big enough to slide out the kidney. The donor usually spends a couple of days in the hospital and, other than athletic exertions I'd shun anyway, can resume normal activities within a week or two. The main dangers are those of any major surgery: general anesthesia, bleeding, infection. They're serious risks, but people go through equally tough operations every day for purely cosmetic reasons.

Contrary to what most people think, living with one kidney is basically the same as living with two. The remaining organ grows to take up the slack. Someone with a single organ is no more vulnerable to kidney failure than someone with a pair, because most kidney disease attacks both at once. The exceptions are injuries, of course, and cancer. I was willing to take my chances.

What about my husband? As I'd expected, he wasn't thrilled with the idea of letting someone slice open his wife, and he was afraid of the tiny but real risk that I might die. He liked Sally but didn't know her that well. He's a rational guy, however, and he knows what sort of person he married. He said okay.

I sent Sally a quick e-mail, confirming that she did in fact need a transplant. She already had a likely prospect, she said. "If your lead doesn't come through, let me know," I wrote back. "If I'm compatible, I'll be a donor." After a couple more exchanges, Sally put me in touch with her transplant coordinator.

The first step to becoming a kidney donor, I discovered, is to give blood – the easiest way to find out your blood type and, conveniently, a great test of squeamishness. My mother had always assured me that I was type O, like her, and thus a universal donor. Yet I didn't even make it to the blood typing. Like many women, I was a shade anemic, with hemoglobin of 12.3

grams per deciliter instead of the required 12.5.

I went into training, eating iron-rich Total cereal for lunch every day. A week later, I hit the magic number, contributed a pint to the Texas blood supply, and a couple days after that, found out my blood type. Bad news: I was A positive, not universally compatible after all. "Will that work?" I e-mailed Sally.

Miraculously, it would. She was also type A, but she didn't expect to need me. I was to be the backup to "Bob from Canada," a guy Sally had found via matching-donors. com, a site for people looking for organ donors. The mysteriously generous Bob was our hero. (My husband was particularly fond of him.)

But in mid-December, Sally suddenly lost touch with him. "I feel like Charlie Brown trying to kick the freaking football and Lucy keeps yanking it away," Sally e-mailed, asking me to get some basic blood and urine tests done in Dallas. By early January Bob was gone. A busy life had interfered with his good intentions.

Soon I was at the Washington Hospital Center, in D.C., filling lots of blood vials to make sure I had no diseases my kidney might pass along. I got an X-ray and an electrocardiogram. On a later trip, I met with a social worker, a nephrologist, and the surgeon, and I had a CT scan to confirm that I really had two healthy kidneys and determine which was the better of the two to take (in my case, the right).

The screening process was peculiarly gratifying. My brothers climb mountains and run marathons, and my parents work out with personal trainers three times a week, which makes me the family couch potato. My primary form of exercise is walking to restaurants. But compared with most would-be kidney donors – the not-so-healthy relatives of very sick people – I was a paragon of fitness: blood pressure on the low end of normal, no hepatitis C, no diabetes, an abdomen that these days passes for slim. (Laparoscopic surgery is more difficult, and sometimes impossible, if the donor is obese.) Everyone at the hospital was impressed. Yea for me!

Most important, it turned out, I had the right personality. Donating a kidney isn't, in fact, a matter of just showing up. You have to be pushy. Unless you're absolutely determined, you'll give up, and nobody will blame you – except, of course, the person who needs a kidney. When I went to see my Dallas doctor for preliminary tests, the first thing she said was, "You know, you can change your mind."

To me, giving Sally a kidney was a practical, straightforward solution to a serious problem. It was important to her but not really a big deal to me. Until the surgery was scheduled – for Saturday, March 4 – and I started telling people about it, I had no idea just how weird I was.

Normal people, I found, have a visceral – pun definitely intended – reaction to the idea of donating an organ. They're revolted. They identify entirely with the donor but not at all with the recipient. They don't compare kidney donation to other risky behavior, like flying a plane or running 31 miles to the bottom of the Grand Canyon and back, as my brother did last summer.

I was scared, of course – but of the surgery, not the loss of my kidney. I'd never been hospitalized before and, except for oral surgery when I was seven, had never had general anesthesia. Surgery, no matter how routine, is dangerous. The kidney is fed by a large renal artery and drained by a large renal vein. If the surgeon cut the wrong one, he'd have five seconds before I bled to death. (I didn't share this tidbit with my husband until after the operation.)

I did my taxes early so my husband wouldn't be stuck sorting through my business receipts if I were incapacitated, or worse. I arranged to stay at a friend's Washington crash pad. I asked the transplant coordinator to tell me, step-by-step, exactly what would happen once I got to the hospital so there would be no surprises.

Things went pretty much as advertised. One minute Sally and I were on beds being wheeled down the hall. I was nervous for about two seconds.

And then I woke up. My husband and parents were there, looking relieved. The nurse took off my oxygen mask so they could feed me ice chips – not too many or I'd throw up. Eventually I moved on to water and clear foods, including tea to fight caffeine withdrawal. Sally had arranged a huge hotel-style room for me, complete with a sofa bed for my husband and real meals. He ate steak while I sipped broth and slurped lime Jell-O.

Yes, I did throw up. Three times and quite violently – a reaction to the anesthesia. I got used to answering a list of excretory questions, starting with "Have you passed gas?" After 24 hours on a catheter, my body refused for a while to urinate on command. When I learned to pee again, the nurse did a victory dance. All in all, it was a very dignified experience.

The worst moment was an early-morning visit by a grave, haggard surgeon – not mine but Sally's. What if Sally had died? What if giving her a kidney had killed her? I'd never seriously considered that possibility.

To my great relief, the surgeon said my friend was okay. But she had had a close call. She'd started hemorrhaging. They'd had to take her back into surgery to stop the bleeding. He'd done hundreds of these operations, and this had never happened. Sally was in intensive care. It had been a very long night.

A day later, when I was off my IV and able to walk-through the hospital, we visited Sally. A tiny woman, she looked like a baby bird, with her short hair shooting up randomly and her skin slightly gray. She was groggy, a bit grouchy, and not entirely coherent. But she knew one thing clearly: "I almost died," she said.

On Tuesday we visited her again before leaving the hospital. She was still in the ICU but about to be moved. She looked like herself. She was talking to friends on her cell phone. What a relief.

Sally left the hospital the following Sunday, the day I had my surgical staples removed. We joined her and a couple of friends for a messy hamburger lunch at her apartment. The next day, we flew home to Dallas.

I never had much pain and, once I left the hospital, took nothing stronger than aspirin, which my surgeon prescribed to prevent blood clots. But it took me about three weeks – longer than I expected – to get back to normal. The surgery had left me easily exhausted. Always a sleepy person, I was taking four-hour naps and falling behind on my deadlines.

Then suddenly I was myself again, with only an occasional twinge in what my husband calls the KV (for "kidney void") to remind me of my medical adventure. I caught up with my work and started traveling – short trips, with light luggage. My all-purpose excuse, "I just donated a kidney," had expired.

On April 10, less than six weeks after the surgery, Sally too went back to work. "I am waiting to be exhausted but I am not... darn," she wrote. "I may be back to normal. Don't think I am nuts but I liked being home and having everyone make a fuss."

She was finally better than before the operation.

Her new kidney was working perfectly, she was no longer anemic, and she no longer had to take five medicines to ward off hypertension. I had never thought much of my kidney when I had it, but now it makes me proud.

She signed the e-mail "Spoiled in D.C."

By Virginia Postrel
(First published in the Texas Monthly. June 2006)
Reprinted by Permission

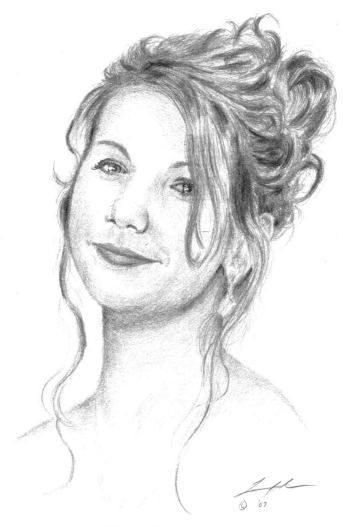

Kari Simmons
Heart Recipient

26

Caring For Kari

By Jan Cunningham (Kari's Mother)

When you give birth, you begin to realize how dramatically a single event can change your life – forever. You also realize how vulnerable you are to events that impact your children's lives. I realized how truly vulnerable we all are on a lovely Memorial Day in 1995. My husband, Danny, and I sat at our dining room table with several neighbors, enjoying the end of the three-day holiday weekend. Waiting for our children to come home from a weekend with their father, Mark, Danny and I laughed and told stories as we watched the neighbors' children play in the front yard.

I knew my 16-year-old daughter, Kari, was not feeling well the minute she walked in the door. Her color was bad, kind of gray. Kari's usually sparkling blue eyes were lifeless. Then I knew things really were bad when her younger brothers told me she had laid on the truck's tailgate while they rode dirt bikes with their dad. She looked very sick, worse than when she left home Friday. She had seemed to have a stomach bug earlier in the week, but we thought she had kicked it.

My sons went off to play with the neighbors and Kari went to her room to lie down. The neighborhood mothers sitting around the table quickly went into consultation mode. These experts agreed it was probably just a stomach bug, but that if Kari weren't better by morning, she should see a doctor.

The night did not go well. Though Kari mostly slept, Danny and I mostly worried. By morning, she looked worse. I got the boys off to school, called in to work and, at 9:00 a.m., phoned the doctor's office. They couldn't see Kari until 4:30 p.m. and couldn't give me a referral to the emergency room based on my explanation of her symptoms. She continued to look bad, was unresponsive and couldn't keep anything down. Becoming impatient and frightened, I knew this was serious, so, with or without a referral, I wasn't waiting until 4:30.

I wrapped Kari up and took her to the emergency room. While I checked her in, the triage nurse started getting Kari's vitals. There were problems with Kari's blood pressure and her heartbeat. They took her back into the E. R. while I finished signing her in. I was alone and scared, but, even worse, Kari was alone and surely she was scared.

I called Danny to tell him that things were pretty bad and that he needed to come to the hospital – now. It seemed like forever until the nurse returned and, when she did, the news was earth-shattering. Kari's heart had quit working correctly. The cause was unknown. She had been stabilized, but they would need to keep her overnight to monitor her. Then there would be consultations with cardiologists and doctors before deciding what to do next.

Kari was tiny, weighing about 100 lbs., but she was not small in attitude. She seemed to feel much better right away and really did not show any signs of being frightened by the news. Her biggest concern was that she had been too sick to wash her hair and now it looked awful. Kari had gorgeous, corn silk-blonde hair that fell straight against her back to her waist.

By the time she got settled into her room, the news of Kari's health crisis had spread at school. Her friends were calling the hospital trying to find her. Although she needed to rest, Kari and her teenage friends managed to talk the nurses and me into letting in a few girls for a short visit. They came armed with beauty aids to help get her through the dirty-hair crisis. They pampered her, fussed over her and cried over her, which really made her feel loved.

The cardiac unit was normally inhabited by the geriatric set, so its staff was not sure how to take the arrival of teens and a mother lioness, which I had become in the few hours we had been there. Kari and her entourage were a novelty for this unit of the hospital and the staff was very attentive. In addition, Kari is one of the sweetest and most polite people in the world, often apologizing to the nurses for being a burden when they were taking care of her.

The cardiologist on duty came to talk to us and explained that Kari's heart muscle was enlarged and her mitral valve was not functioning properly. More testing was required. The medical team decided to move Kari to Children's Mercy Hospital in downtown Kansas City, Mo., because that facility would be better equipped to deal with a child of her age facing such a problem. I had always known that Children's Mercy had an incredible reputation and that if any of the kids ever had a serious health problem I would want them treated there.

At Children's Mercy, Kari got settled in a room, and was hooked up to all the latest gadgetry and stabilized. I had not slept the night before and, once Kari was settled in, the nursing staff and Carmie – Kari's "other mom" and mother of her long-time friend, Jeannette, convinced me to go home for the night. Carmie would stay with Kari until she was asleep, which made me feel better. I was reluctant to leave but had three boys at home who needed supervision.

After I had been home a few hours, I laid down and quickly fell asleep. About 20 minutes later the phone rang. It was a nurse at Children's Mercy, calling to tell me that Kari had become unstable and disoriented, and had been moved to the ICU. I found out very quickly that, with the right motivation, a Chevy minivan can fly. In 15 minutes, I had called my husband, gotten dressed, flown down I-35, parked illegally at Children's Mercy and was standing next to Kari's ICU bed at the hospital. On that seven-minute drive, I vowed to never leave Kari alone in the hospital again.

She was stable and awake. She told me she knew who and where she was, but that the staff had awakened her and she couldn't tell them the answers they wanted to hear. It was clear that she was disoriented.

Danny and I kept company that night and over the next few days with other parents, all sharing their stories and fighting for their children's lives. There were never any fights with the doctors or nurses, just the fight we all had taken on against the evil that would try to harm our innocent children.

We were surrounded by extremely sad stories, but the attitudes of everyone in the hospital were hopeful and positive. Over the days that followed, Kari went through many tests and we all learned more about heart function than we ever dreamed possible. Kari was diagnosed with dilated cardiomyopathy and mitral valve prolapse caused by a virus that attacked her heart muscle. Doctors believed they could manage her condition with medication and, over the next few days, worked to get her medication regulated so that she could get back home and back to her life.

We were finally discharged from the hospital with several prescriptions and a follow-up appointment in the cardiology clinic. No one ever said it and it was quite awhile before I asked, but I knew that, eventually, Kari would need a new heart. For now though, she was fine.

Kari managed to finish her junior year of high school without too much problem. She completed a course of cardiac rehabilitation and became active with Children's Mercy's Heart Camp. She had a couple of instances of a trial fibrillation which required that she be cardio-verted but, all in all, that first year went pretty well.

Her senior year was not as easy. Kari was very active in her school's drama department, classes were hectic and being a teen is hard when you are tired and sick most of the time. Kari was named homecoming queen and graduated from high school. The a-fib episodes increased and she was cardio-verted numerous times throughout the year. Each time the procedure got harder on her and her heart would not stay in rhythm as long.

By September, Kari had decided to begin classes at Johnson County Community College while she figured out what she wanted to do long-term. The first semester came to an end early for her, however. Cardio-version was not a permanent fix for the atrial fibrillation and, after two more attempts, we were told that Kari was in congestive heart failure.

I had never dreamed this day would come so quickly. I thought we had 15 years before a transplant would be necessary. We had put a lot of hope in the idea that something would be discovered that would help her before she had to have a transplant. But the discovery never came and Kari's window of opportunity was closing.

The doctors at Children's Mercy decided that, due to her age, it was time to move Kari to another hospital. Also, if she were evaluated for transplant at a children's hospital she would have to go to St. Louis or Minnesota for the transplant. Although she was stable, her condition continued to deteriorate. We had grown very close to the staff at Children's Mercy and had a great deal of trust in their knowledge and recommendations, so we weren't excited about changing hospitals and trying to adjust to new doctors at such a critical time, but it was the best answer for Kari.

She was transported by ambulance to St. Luke's Hospital and checked into one of the transplant rooms. We met with the transplant nurse coordinator and the transplant cardiologist, Dr. Janet Stephens, who had been recommended by the cardiologist at Children's Mercy. Dr. Stephens was extremely kind and thoroughly explained the process to us.

Kari would go through a long series of evaluations that included blood work, a dental evaluation, a gynecological evaluation and a psychiatric evaluation. Before the evaluations began, we learned that our insurance would not cover Dr. Stephens' group and we would have to use a doctor from another group on staff at the hospital. We were introduced to Dr. Genton and his transplant nurse coordinator. Dr. Genton was very kind and gentle, and immediately was enamored by Kari's charms and she his. Elaine, the nurse coordinator, was an energetic mother figure that I felt instantly I could trust.

They discussed again the evaluation process and the waiting process, and how Kari could manage the congestive heart failure while she waited. Each doctor we met made sure we understood fully that a transplant was not a cure, but simply a solution she could live with. The congestive heart failure would kill her; the transplant was her only hope. But we had to understand, too, that there are serious side effects with the post-transplant medication and that Kari would have to manage her medication and pay strict attention to her health.

The hospital's transplant support system also kicked into action. Kari had numerous visits by transplant recipients who were members of the support group *Heartline*. They helped her understand what was ahead and answered her questions. Most of the *Heartline* members were older, in their 50s and 60s, but Kari developed a relationship with each of them.

The evaluations were finally completed. Kari had to have her wisdom teeth removed before she could be placed on the list, but otherwise was approved for the transplant. Her wisdom teeth were extracted in the hospital in case there were any complications due to her weakened condition. By that time, it was late November and the doctors said she was strong enough to go home, with a pager, to wait for the call. We had to be ready at a moment's notice. We could get the call that day or it could be months, but at least there was hope.

Kari was young and very small, and most people on

the list are larger and older. I think that is when the brutal reality hit me – someone else's child would have to die for Kari to live. I knew this but it had not hit home until that moment, at least not that it would be someone else's child. Of course, I knew that we were not choosing for someone to die. We knew that, when it inevitably happened, it would be perhaps the only positive outcome to another child's untimely death.

Kari waited patiently at home, but swiftly became extremely weak and was retaining fluids badly. She was hospitalized for short periods during her waiting time, but the doctors never wanted her there for long – there was too much flu and sickness in the hospital and she needed to be healthy when a heart became available.

While we waited for Kari's new heart, we were moved by the outreach and support people offered. Our friends, family and co-workers set up a "Care for Kari" campaign to help raise money to defray the immense costs we would incur. Although I had very good insurance, there was no doubt that we would have extraordinary medical bills from the transplant in addition to those we had already incurred during her illness. People were not just concerned about her health and well being, but also about the financial impact the transplant would have on our family. A trust fund was started for her with the proceeds from the fundraisers. The outpouring of love, concern and empathy with her situation and our pain as her parents was heart-wrenching.

I had been very active in my employer's community service program, but had never been on the receiving end. It occurs to me now that making a donation to a cause is much easier than being the recipient. It is very humbling to be in a vulnerable situation, to be in need.

This was a time when our entire family had to put our pride behind us and accept help. Financial and emotional help were greatly appreciated, but the focus of our prayers was on the donation of a lifetime, the donation of life itself for Kari.

Everyone was on edge at our house over the next months. If the phone rang we jumped. Kari's pager went off a couple of times, but it turned out to be wrong numbers. Kari's condition continued to deteriorate. She had good days and bad but, for the most part, would be worn out walking from her room to the bathroom. She stayed downstairs most of the day and watched out the window. Her color was very gray and her eyes once again lacked their sparkle.

On Friday, March 20, 1998, Kari was feeling well enough to go watch a church volleyball game. She had grown quite stir crazy, but didn't often have the strength or inclination to go out. Danny and I were just winding down and recapping the week's activities when Elaine, the transplant nurse coordinator, called and asked for Kari. I thought Elaine's voice seemed more excited than usual. I asked her if a heart was available and she said, "I need to talk to Kari. Does she have her pager with her?" I told her she did and asked again if this meant they had found a heart. All she would say is that it looked like there might be one but not to get too excited until we found out for sure and could be certain the match was good.

Only minutes after Elaine hung up, Kari called, wondering if I had heard the news. She said that she was on her way home to get ready to go to the hospital, but that she had a little time since the surgery was not yet certain.

When Kari came in, everyone was excited and a bit worried. The waiting had been terrible so far. She was not out of the woods yet and we all knew many things could go wrong. None of us focused on the 'what ifs;' we concentrated on the 'maybe.' Danny and I were busily making phone calls and trying to get together the things we might need at the hospital when we realized that Kari was sitting on the floor hugging Buster, our 110-lb. golden retriever, and crying.

She had rarely cried throughout her ordeal and I had been forbidden to cry in front of her. We spent a little time hugging, crying and talking about her mixture of joy, fear and apprehension. It didn't take long for us to get back on track, and remember we had an important appointment and we needed to get to St. Luke's.

When we arrived, Elaine met us with the news that Kari would be prepped, but they still were not certain whether the surgery would happen. Kari's entourage already had started to amass. There was a lot of energy and faith in the room, not to mention noise.

Along two walls were curtained areas – kind of a staging area outside the cardiac O. R. – with several people waiting to go into surgery. Against the other two walls were surgical ICU suites, one of which Kari would be moved into for a few days following the surgery. In the center of the room was a big nurse's station with all of the monitoring equipment, charts and other mysterious tools of the trade. It was a beehive of activity. Kari wasn't alone in the center of it, but she was the center of our attention.

The evening crept along. Family and friends stuck close by Kari all evening, keeping her mind occupied and her spirits up while we waited. The medical staff finally gave Kari something to relax and she started getting silly. Kari did not cope well with drugs and was pretty funny to watch. Her dad even got quite a few laughs for his attempts at jokes. After what seemed like forever, the doctors came out and said that the surgery was a go. Another transplant recipient had just been taken back also. These would be the first simultaneous heart transplants performed at St. Luke's.

The staff wheeled Kari down the long hall and through the O. R. doors at around 11:30 p.m. We were sent to the waiting room, where we stayed with a large group of friends and family waiting for news of Kari. Sadly, other families were in the waiting room also — families whose joy was being taken away while we were being given hope again.

I remember friends trying to get me to eat. I remember trying to sleep. I remember trying to keep the gang quiet and keep my wits about me. I don't remember how long Kari was gone, how long the surgery took or what time they came to tell us that she was in recovery and that things had gone very well, but I will never forget the way Kari looked when I was finally allowed to see her. She was so helpless lying there, still sedated from the surgery. She was naked except for a sheet barely covering her. There were tubes and wires, and her body seemed so small and helpless. What had they done to my beautiful little girl? There was an eight-inch incision down her chest between her breasts. One thing occurred to me instantly though: She was pink again. Her color had already started to come back and, while she looked pretty frightening, she looked so much better.

The doctors and nurses seemed to go out of their way to make sure Kari kept a positive attitude. Their care was extraordinary throughout the 11 days we were at the hospital. Visits from other transplant recipients helped ease the anxiety of the new addition to her body. She longed to go home, to drive, and to get out and about with friends. We were somewhat apprehensive about her susceptibility to disease and infection when she came home.

We were given several training sessions on her pharmaceutical regimen, which at one point included up to 17 tablets throughout the day. Thank goodness the medical staff wrote it down in a notebook for us. The doctors had done an excellent job bringing complete life back to our angel.

In preparation for Kari's homecoming, her friends Jeanette and Shelly came to the house and thoroughly cleaned her room. I began taking daily tours of the house with Clorox and rubber gloves, wiping down doorknobs, light switches, handrails and anything else that someone might touch or breathe on. Diligent hand washing became more critical than ever.

The day finally came when she was allowed to come home. Kari donned her mask and was loaded into a wheelchair for the trip to the car.

Following each clinic visit, we would await the 1:00 p.m. phone call the following day to tell us that Kari was a zero, no rejection. The fear of rejection lessened with each visit. We went from weekly visits, to monthly, then every three months, then every six months. Then the annual visit. Eventually, Kari told me that I didn't need to go to the clinic with her anymore.

At almost ten years post-transplant, Kari continues to thrive. She is a medical assistant at her cardiologist's office. A vital and active young woman, she is involved in her church, busy with friends, and trying to buy and rehab an older house. Kari also plays an active role in the lives of her two nieces, Ciaran and Stylee, sharing her love of life and herself with them unselfishly. Most recently, Kari has given her heart in a different way and has married an amazing man, Chuck, who loves her wholly. She has also been given the privilege of being a step-mom to Chaz, an equally amazing boy.

Kari has a strong respect for life and the gift she has been given. She has seen many friends from her transplant group pass away from complications and from natural causes. She sees friends who are healthy and take it for granted. She knows that each day is possible because of the gift of life given to her by someone she never knew.

I often think of how the transplant and illness changed her life and our entire family, but I try to never think of how our lives would have been had she been taken from us.

* * *

Our Family's Tribute and Gratitude

Our Kari would have died, there is no doubt, had a heart not become available in time. The devastation our family would have suffered is unfathomable. While we all believed that organ donation was important and was the decision we would make if ever faced with the choice, we now know first hand the impact it can have on a life and a family. Each of us has made a concerted effort to encourage others to understand organ donation and be able to make that choice, sign the donor information on driver's licenses and ensure that the family understands the desire to donate organs in the case of death.

After Kari's transplant, both she and I tried numerous times to write a letter that would be delivered to the donor family via the organ donor bank. Saying thank you isn't hard, it just didn't seem like enough.

We were always at a loss for words, never able to express the heartfelt gratitude in such bittersweet circumstances. Kari received her transplant on the first day of spring. It was new life and new beginnings for us, but a painful winter for another family. Avoiding any more pain for them was our main concern.

We always felt that we knew where the heart had come from, but were not 100 percent certain. Our community is not that large and it seemed that we had friends in common with the donor family. It was not until October of Kari's sixth year post-transplant, however, that we were able to make contact, and it came about in a rather miraculous way.

Kari's stepfather, Dan, was passing time talking with an acquaintance, Ray, at a farmer's market. The men had known each other casually for some time but did not know each other well. Ray had sold vegetables to Dan on a weekly basis during the summer months and Dan occasionally brought Ray homemade bread to return the favor.

The subject of sick children came up, and Dan mentioned in passing that his daughter Kari had some very serious health problems but had been saved because of a heart transplant. Ray mentioned that he lost a daughter, Keeley, a few years earlier and that, although the decision was difficult, the family had donated her organs. The two men continued to talk, slowly putting together the pieces of the puzzle.

As the picture became clearer, both men came to realize that Keeley's heart had been transplanted into Kari. Keeley's death had allowed Kari to go on living. While standing in the middle of the farmer's market, the two men lost control of their emotions and embraced, crying. No longer just casual acquaintances, they now had an unbreakable bond that soon would become a deep relationship. This chance meeting between acquaintances was just the first meeting between the two families.

Because of the courageous decision made by Keeley's parents, we were able to meet the most incredible, selfless people on the planet – and they have become important members of our extended family. The greatest honor was having them at Kari's wedding. We will always be thankful to them for their selfless gift. In honor of the beautiful, smiling, giggling Keeley, we have our story to tell. Keeley's heart now beats in our daughter, Kari.

Keeley was 13 years old when she suffered a seizure and died. She had been in a wheelchair all of her life because she suffered from cerebral palsy. Although we never met Keeley, she will always be an integral part of our lives. And, as her obituary read – and I truly believe – she is free of her wheelchair and is walking with God.

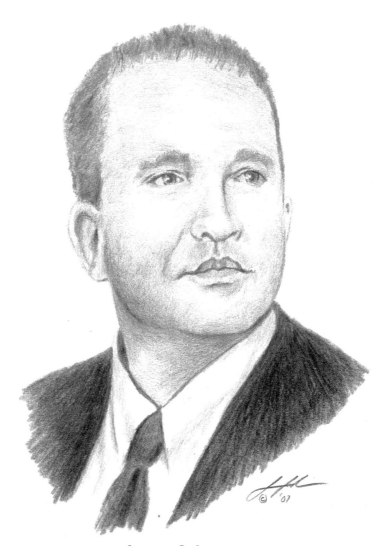

Aaron Schurman
Kidney Recipient

27

A Life With Kidney Problems
By Aaron Schurman

My name is Aaron and, by the grace of God, I am here today to share with you my hope and fears, strength and experience about kidney transplants. I will tell you about how it felt going through the tests, the waiting, and the events leading up to, during and after the transplant.

Hannah Moore once said, "Obstacles are those frightful things you see when you take your eyes off your goal." Each of us has a choice to make when we are challenged by adversity and we have to overcome the obstacles that are put in our paths. We can be overcome by them, whine about them and feel sorry for ourselves about them – and thus diminish the quality of our lives. Or, we can see those challenges as opportunities to learn and grow, accepting them peacefully and using our experience to help others, thus enhancing the quality of our lives and giving hope to others in the process.

There is a story about an older man who, day after day, slowly walked the beaches by the ocean, carefully, one by one, picking up some of the thousands of starfish that had washed onto shore and throwing them back into the sea. Every day he did this at the same time a young lady was jogging along the beach. Curious about the man's purpose, she finally stopped and asked why he would waste his time and energy bending over and throwing these starfish back into the ocean. She said to him, "There are thousands of them. You really can't think you are making much of a difference, can you?" The man gently bent over one more time, picked up another starfish and threw it back into the ocean. He said to the young lady, "It just made a difference to that one."

These stories illustrate the power of perception, which is how we view, see or look at someone or something. Perception determines our attitudes, which reflect how we feel about someone or something. Those who perceive positively usually feel and act positively. Those who perceive negatively usually feel and act negatively. It is the power of choice. And that is what I want to talk to you about today.

Each of us is where we are and who we are because of our choices and our experiences. Since I was 12, I have made many choices. Some of them were life-threatening and others were life-saving. I would like to share my story with you. It is a story that I trust will be inspiring and give hope to those who are struggling with major health issues.

I grew up on a Nebraska farm with my parents and two older sisters. I led what I thought was a normal life during my first 12 years. I was small for my age, but so was my older sister until she entered high school, so I wasn't worried. I figured we were all just "slow growers." When I was about 10, I began to lack energy, always feeling tired, and didn't want to do things that most young boys do. The doctor's visits were frequent, as were the tests to determine the cause of my fatigue. While in eighth grade I was referred to Dr. Thomas Knight, a nephrologist at Clarkson Hospital in Omaha, for extensive testing. After going through several tests I began to realize that something serious could be wrong. The hospital did a kidney biopsy, placing a needle in my back and taking a very small sample of one of my kidneys.

I'm glad that, as a youngster, I was so naivë about what was happening medically. I think that, if I had been an adult, it would have been much scarier. As it was, I had no clue what was going on in my body and had many questions. Why did this happen to me? Did I do something to make this happen? Does anyone else in our family have a history of kidney disease? Am I going to die? Of course, my parents didn't want to elaborate on anything to scare me any more than I already was, but they, too, had no idea of the road we would be taking, or where or when it would come to an end.

Dr. Knight diagnosed me with a kidney disease called "membranoproliferative glomerulonephritis, Type 1." This meant that my kidneys were failing and I would have to undergo a kidney transplant at some future date. I remember feeling the fear and anxiety about what my future would be like, or if I even would have a future. I remember leaving the hospital and going out for pizza with my family. We tried to act as if nothing had changed, like this never happened, yet I felt sure that my life was never going to be the same again.

I was prescribed medications and routinely had tests to make sure my kidneys weren't failing too fast.

During my junior year in high school, I took the next

medical step. I would have to go on dialysis because my kidneys were failing. I had surgery to place a dialysis tube in my stomach so I could hook up to the machine that would clean my blood. I was hooked up to that machine every night for eight hours. I hated what was happening to me. This wasn't what high school juniors were supposed to be doing at night.

I was placed on a transplant list, which required a variety of tests. My mother took the initial blood work to see if she might be a possible match for me. She qualified as a possible donor and proceeded with the rest of the testing process. After a couple of months, she found out she could give me one of her kidneys, which she decided to do without hesitation.

The surgery took place after about four months of dialysis. I came through that surgery in good condition. Several of my family and friends even commented that I looked healthier than I had in a long time. It is amazing how fast the skin color returns after a transplant. Within a couple of hours, my skin changed from a pale white to a pinkish color.

I knew how fortunate I was immediately after surgery, but, less than a month later, there were complications. The first was a blood clot that formed in my leg, requiring surgery. After about a week, it was obvious that the initial surgery to deal with the clot didn't work, so I had to have a second surgery. This time, the surgeon accidentally nicked the new kidney and it stopped functioning completely. You can imagine my family's thoughts and emotions. "Did we just lose everything we worked for in two seconds?"

The doctors fixed the damage after a couple of days and hoped, like I did, that the kidney wouldn't fail during the next few days or weeks. I had several tests to check for damage.

I was then placed on dialysis for a couple of days to try to reverse the damage that had been done and to get the kidney functioning well again.

Looking back with the benefit of hindsight, I don't think I was as grateful as I should have been about my kidney transplant. After all, I was just 17 years old, and I would rather have been doing other things in my life. Going through a transplant requires commitment, trust, determination and the patience to heal. My mother sacrificed a great deal for me and, at the time, I didn't really show her the kind of appreciation she deserved. Mom had her kidney removed by the 'open' procedure, which is more difficult than the laparoscopic technique commonly used now. The healing time for her was several months, compared to about one month with today's procedure. This shows truly how great a mother's love is. Today, she knows how exceptionally grateful I am for her love and support.

During the next seven years of my life, I went to school, worked and lived an active life. I still had to deal with the fear of my kidney failing, going through another transplant and having dialysis again but, for the most part, I got on with my life and coped pretty well. One of the greatest obstacles I had to face was not physical but mental. I fought through surgeries time and time again, but the one thing that bothered me was that, in my mind, I was not a normal human being with a healthy body and that getting into a relationship with anyone was not for me. I had very low perception of myself and didn't want to have a girlfriend that would have to deal with my health problems. I actually thought there wasn't anyone out there who would want to date a transplant recipient. This was something I had to work at for a very long time and, at times, still sits in the back of my mind.

Sometime during my seventh year after transplant, I began to experience kidney failure. The cause was unknown. I felt powerless because I could do nothing to stop it. I knew I wasn't to blame, yet wondered if something I did had triggered it. I was very scared because I knew the path I had traveled the first time to get to this point and refused to ever go down it again. I made up my mind to avoid and ignore my doctors, and to not get lab work done to monitor my kidney.

Deep inside I knew I was being irresponsible about my health. I think it was just that I was fearful, and sick and tired of dealing with all of the medical stuff. I got calls from the medical staff at Clarkson Hospital, asking me to get my lab work done and get my kidney checked. I usually hung up on them and made a vow that I would not deal with a transplant again. This went on for about two years until one day, I finally changed my mind.

I went back to Clarkson for tests to see what damage had been done to my kidney. It turned out that the kidney was barely functioning and that I needed to go back on dialysis. I hated doing this, but knew that if I wanted to live I would have to stay with the program my doctors believed would work for me. So, I stayed faithful, getting tests regularly and keeping up with my dialysis.

To make matters worse, I chose not to tell my parents, thinking that the news of the kidney failing would "disappoint" them and that they may think differently of me for having to go through dialysis again. The only reason they found out was because my mom became suspicious and called one of the hospital's transplant coordinators.

To start the dialysis process again, doctors inserted a temporary access site in my neck until they could surgically place the permanent tube in my stomach cavity. I was immediately put on hemodialysis, a form of dialysis where I was placed on a machine for three to four hours a day, three days a week. This form of dialysis is very draining and gave me flu-like symptoms every time. I continued this treatment for about two months until the permanent tube was placed in my stomach.

To continue hemodialysis full time requires a permanent access site in one's arm. I had the surgery to place a tube in my stomach for a different type of dialysis that I could do at home instead of going to a center every three days. After the tube in my stomach healed, I started home dialysis four times daily, continuing this for the next three years.

The home dialysis, called peritoneal dialysis, went pretty well for about a year. The longer a person is on dialysis, the greater the chance problems will develop. One of the first problems I experienced was difficulty eating or drinking anything without being in extreme pain afterward. My body simply couldn't digest the food and it would just sit in my stomach, a condition known as pancreatitis. Before being diagnosed correctly, I went to the emergency room three times, was given strong painkillers and sent home. This was very frustrating and discouraging.

About a week after the third trip to the emergency room, I had a very painful pancreatitis episode and knowingly doubled my medication dosage to try to stop the pain. I had been passed out on my bed for a day when my parents called my apartment. I was very incoherent.

Concerned and scared, they called 911. They live about 60 miles from me and must have felt powerless. The ambulance arrived and took me to the emergency room for the fourth time. During this trip, doctors finally confirmed that I had pancreatitis. I immediately went through surgery to remove my gall bladder, the cause of the painful episodes. I was in the hospital this time for two weeks and couldn't take any food or water, just liquids from intravenous feedings.

During the next year of my life, my health took a turn for the worse again. I learned that, because of the length of time on dialysis, my problems likely would become more frequent. I got nerve damage in my feet and legs when the dialysis failed to pull enough fluid from my body, and the excess fluid went to my feet and legs, causing swelling. After a month of the swelling, there was enough nerve damage that I walked like I was a 95-year-old person.

By this time, I had been on the transplant list for approximately a year and a half, knowing that the average wait time for my blood type was close to five years. Since I was on dialysis for so long, my blood had a very high phosphorous level, causing me to itch constantly, like I had poison ivy. It also can cause other complications, so the doctors decided to take out my parathyroid gland to lower the phosphorous levels in my blood. I checked into Bryan Hospital in Lincoln for this surgery. I already had lost 30 pounds, and was getting thin and weak. Time was running out to find a suitable donor.

I swore to my family that I would not allow any of them to donate again, even if they were a match. I had seen what it had done to my mother and didn't want anyone to go through that again. In spite of this, my Uncle Tom was getting tested without my knowledge. It turned out that he was close to a match but had some things to work out before it would become a reality. Both of us went through thorough testing. The first major obstacle was to take out my old, failed kidney to see if that would improve the way we matched.

During this time, other family complications made life ever more difficult, as we watched my Grandmother pass away two days before the surgery. I felt sad, discouraged and angry about what was happening, but I had to have the surgery instead of going to the funeral.

It was a brutal and painful surgery. The doctors had to remove the kidney from an area filled with scar tissue from previous surgeries. The surgery resulted in neck and back problems for me for at least the next six months. I could barely walk and lost an additional 10 pounds. My health was getting worse, not better.

The day after surgery – one of the scariest moments in my life – I woke up and could hardly breathe. I called the doctors and described the symptoms, and they determined that I had too much fluid in my lungs. Numerous people surrounded me, all in panic mode. It became harder and harder to breathe. I honestly thought I was going to die on the same day as my Grandmother's funeral. It took a long time to recover from this surgery, both mentally and physically. In fact, some of my family and friends would tell you that I was never the same after that surgery. Less than a month later, Tom and I had a positive cross-match; he was no longer a compatible donor.

I wanted to give up and wished that the whole kidney problem and dialysis would just go away. I am a very strong person mentally, but everyone has a breaking point and mine was very close. The reality of the situation was not going away and the past year-and-a-half of testing with Tom was now gone. It was depressing, discouraging and very disappointing.

In January 2002, my sister, Michelle, came to visit me in Lincoln and shared some uplifting news. Without my knowledge, she had gotten the initial lab work and learned she might be a suitable kidney donor. She went behind my back to get tested because she knew that I didn't need a transplant 'someday' – I needed one now. She asked me if I would accept a kidney from her. I could not answer her question on the spot; I waited about a week before I allowed her to continue with the testing. I was bound and determined to not let another family member go through surgery, but I had very limited choices. I knew it was a gift that couldn't be thrown away. Michelle continued with the testing, completing what normally takes three or four months in far less time. (It didn't hurt that she worked across the street from the hospital.)

I didn't think I could have anymore 'major' problems before the surgery, but I was wrong and soon was challenged again. Due to the surgery to remove my gallbladder, the phosphorus levels in my blood now had become dangerously low, creating a complication that could have ended my life in one night. I fell asleep on a Tuesday night about 10:00 p.m. and woke up on what I thought was Wednesday morning. It turned out to be Thursday afternoon. I had had a seizure while I was sleeping. The doctors weren't sure why I woke up because most people who have seizures in their sleep don't wake up again. Due to the seizure, I developed pneumonia in my right lung and very easily could have drowned in the fluid that collected there.

I believe that only divine intervention has allowed me to be here today. The reason I woke up was because of Scott, the delivery driver from Baxter Home Medical Supplies. Scott thought it would be okay to deliver my supplies a day earlier than planned because he was in the neighborhood anyway. He knocked on the door several times but didn't get an answer. He left, but came back later. He knocked again, loudly enough to wake me. I somehow made it to the door.

Scott noticed right away that I was incoherent and that something was very wrong. He called the Dialysis Center and told them what he saw. Jean, a nurse at the

Dialysis Center, called me and told me to get medical attention right away.

I began to realize that something was really wrong because I didn't know how to get to a hospital and wasn't even sure of my address or name. I was very disoriented, but somehow drove six miles to the hospital. About the only thing I remember was that I got lost driving to a hospital in a town I had lived in for about eight years and that I stopped four or five times because I was unable to stay awake. It took me more than two hours to drive six miles.

Testing confirmed that I had had the seizure and that I had pneumonia in my right lung. I spent the next two weeks in the hospital getting healthy enough to have my transplant in April.

My second transplant was scheduled for April 2, 2002. As if life possibly could become any more frustrating, another test was thrown at our family. A few weeks before the transplant, my mother was diagnosed with breast cancer. Her surgery would be around the same time Michelle and I would have surgery.

Of the five members of our immediate family, three of us were hospitalized for major surgery. To this day I have no idea how my Dad and my other sister, Marie, dealt with the stress of everything that occurred in such a short period.

It seemed like the longest wait of my life, but April 2 had arrived. I met my family in the waiting room around 5:30 a.m. We all sat together until it came time for my sister and me to be prepped for surgery. Michelle was called to prep for surgery at 7:30 a.m.; this was about an hour later than expected. As Michelle left the waiting room, we didn't hug each other or say a word. Prior to the surgery, Michelle and I talked every night on the phone for an hour or more and, at this point, we both knew how we felt, and no exchange was needed.

The rest of us waited in a small, private waiting room to talk and pass the time reading and watching television. Some of my family wanted to talk about the surgery, but I was too nervous and emotional to do that. I had waited for more than three years for this day and it wasn't really sinking in just how much my life was going to change.

About 10:00 a.m., I was given instructions to meet someone to prep me for surgery. It was truly an emotional time. About 20 family members were there, and we exchanged hugs, tears and words of hope. At that moment, when I realized I was going to get the transplant I needed, all of the emotions of the past three years came to the surface.

The surgeries went well for my sister and me, and the kidney started working immediately. Michelle managed to heal fast enough to go back to work in three weeks.

I was in the intensive care unit about three days, was in good spirits and everything seemed to be going well. About a week later, though, I began to experience some of the same problems I had had after the first transplant.

Fluid in my leg caused my leg to swell and I gained more than 10 pounds in fluid overnight. The doctors treated the problem a little differently this time, inserting drainage tubes around the transplanted kidney. One tube was placed in my left side, and I was told I would be going home with it in and that I could empty the drainage bag myself every day. This worked well for about a week, until the tube got plugged and I couldn't drain it anymore. I went back to Clarkson Hospital for further treatment. The doctors, who soon noticed that the tube had moved, decided to remove it and start over.

I was frustrated and discouraged. I reluctantly decided to go ahead, even though the surgery, while not major, was a painful event I didn't want to go through again. The new drainage tube lasted about as long as the first one did before it, too, became plugged and quit draining. Again, I went back to Clarkson to be monitored for the amount of drainage still contained around the kidney. After a couple of days there, the fluid increased so much that my leg, back and chest began to fill. All of what I was going through seemed like a nightmare. It turned out the only doctor on staff that night was a liver specialist who knew little about kidney transplants. He gave me a shot of pain medication, which turned out to be a form of medication that could have caused the kidney to reject. Luckily, it had no ill effect on my kidney.

The following day, my doctors told me I would need a kidney biopsy to determine if my kidney was rejecting. My lab numbers were starting to fall out of the "normal" range, indicating a possible rejection. I thought to myself, "What else could go wrong?" I was beginning to wonder if all of this was worth it. There was also the fear that, during the biopsy, doctors might nick the kidney like before. No one wanted the new kidney to be touched.

Before the biopsy, my lead surgeon told me he thought the kidney was rejecting, but that we would have definite results in about a day. He then said that he would need to insert a second tube into my side during the surgery. I was upset with this choice and argued with him to do the same procedure that had been done 10 years ago. My other doctors first refused to do this surgery, but a few days later agreed to proceed as the lead surgeon directed.

It was the longest 24 hours of my life and of my family's. Did we come this far to now lose everything? Would I reject the kidney and be placed on dialysis again?

Thankfully, I learned the good news the next day that the kidney was not rejecting, but that the lab numbers were higher because the fluid in my body was putting pressure on the kidney. I was treated for a few more days as the fluid decreased and safely drained, then I was released from the hospital with two tubes and two drainage bags on my side that would have to stay there for about a month.

Both of the tubes worked correctly for the first week or so. Shortly after, I woke up one night with fluid in my leg once again, and I could feel massive amounts all the way up into my back and chest. I had so much fluid retention that I couldn't bend at the waist to get out of bed and I had a hard time breathing. It scared me. I managed to get through until morning, when my Dad drove me to the hospital.

I had developed an infection around the kidney and was running a temperature of more than 103 degrees. The doctors took me to surgery immediately to clean out the infection around the kidney because they knew I could lose the kidney if this wasn't done successfully. During the next few days, I was constantly sick to my stomach. The doctors put a tube down into my stomach to try to get the remaining infection out of my system. After about three days, the doctors determined that the infection was gone and removed the tube.

During the first month after my transplant, I lost more than 40 pounds and was left physically weak and emotionally exhausted. I was now down to 108 pounds, looking drawn and skinny. I was confined to the house and had to have daily visits by a home nurse to change the dressing and clean the incision where doctors went in for the second surgery. It took more than five months for the incision to heal and all of the fluid to stop drain-ing. I had to make monthly visits to the hospital in

Omaha for lab work, but I never had to be admitted to the hospital again during those five-months.

This second transplant challenged every bit of my energy and will. There were so many times I just wanted to give up. Someone once told me that 80 percent of life is just showing up. I have to make a correction to that. My life is normal and healthy because my family showed up 100 percent. My mom and sister did the hard part; I just showed up. Without the support of my entire family and numerous people I don't even know, my life could be totally different.

Almost five years have now passed. I have had more than four years of complete health with no complications. Not a day goes by where I don't think about the past and how it has affected the future. A Danish philosopher, Soren Kierkegaard, once said, "Life can be understood backwards, but it must be lived forward." Everyone has things in the past that can be understood differently. I see the roadmap of scars from surgeries I have had and they mean something very important to me. They are there simply to remind me that the past was real.

As I look back at everything that has happened, it's very clear to me that life is lived one day at a time. I am very thankful for the help and support of family and friends and I live my life trying to help other people that also need support. I give what I can to others to try to make their lives a little better. Sometimes it works, sometimes it doesn't. No regrets.

I hope that my story has influenced you in someway. I hope you take from this story that there are real life heroes out there in this world. This story is dedicated to the heroes in my life.

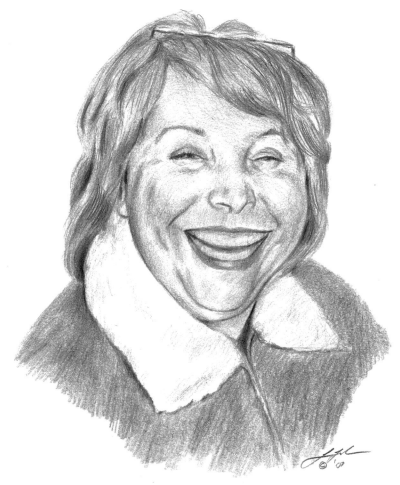

Jean Reyes de Gonzales
Tissue Recipient

28

A Gift Given – and Received

By Jean Reyes de Gonzalez

Hello, my name is Jean Reyes de Gonzalez, and I am here from Connecticut.

In the month of July 2000, I was diagnosed with having a severe problem with a herniated disk in my neck. I had had symptoms for years, but never knew I had a problem.

I would wake up in the night and my left arm would feel tingly, and I would think I must have just slept on it and now it was waking up. I ignored it.

One fateful day I woke up and my arm was hurting, and as the day went on, the pain became more severe. By two o'clock in the afternoon I was carrying my arm because letting it hang was just so painful, I could not tolerate it.

I called my medical plan. They have a twenty-four hour hotline, and if you have not decided whether or not to go to the doctor, you can speak to a triage nurse.

After listening to me she said, "You can wait and make an appointment to see a doctor, but if your arm swells, I would recommend you go to the Emergency Room."

Well, the next morning I woke up and my entire arm was swollen, not just my hand. So I went to the Emergency Room. The doctor in the Emergency Room took x-rays and said, "I think you have a pinched nerve, but I would recommend you go see a neurosurgeon."

That scared me because in my mind, neurosurgery went with brain surgery and I didn't want to have my brain operated on. But I listened to the doctor and I went to the neurosurgeon who then prescribed another series of tests to find out what was the actual cause of this pain.

He told me that I had a herniated disk in the neck and that it was severe enough to require surgery.

They would have to remove the disk. They would have to transplant a piece of bone. They would have to put in a plate with screws to keep my neck together. And that was the plan.

So, when I went home, I was really upset about the whole thing. Just the thought of having surgery, the thought of having neck surgery upset me. I had visions of you know, what if the knife slips? Then he severs my spinal cord instead of repairing it.

All kinds of things went running through my mind.

But, there was a man who had died a couple of months before. His name was John Anthony Amato. He was not able to give his organs because he had actually died at home and was then moved to the Emergency Room.

His wife decided to donate tissue so his corneas

were donated and bone was donated. And his bones were going through the process of being prepared for transplantation.

When it was my turn to receive my bone, the bone bank was notified and John's bone was selected.

I know for a fact that John's wife struggled immensely with going through the process of tissue donation. And therefore I want to thank every family that is here for the courage to not only make the decision 'yes, I want my loved one to live on through donation' but for enduring the process of answering the social questions, the medical history, all required to be able to go through the process so that your loved ones organs could be donated.

She struggled because they had been married for two years and six months and one day, and he had been the love of her life.

She had a difficult childhood and had gone through relationships that had ended because of physical and emotional abuse. When she met John, there was such a dramatic change in her life and she knew for the first time what it meant to be loved unconditionally.

He was the kind of person who was so romantic that he would wake up in the morning and roll over in bed and say, "Hi gorgeous."

He just made her feel so special.

Perhaps you are wondering why I know so much about his wife.

That would be because John Anthony Amato was my husband. He had died in the month of May. He had died of an aortic aneurism at home. We never knew him to be sick, but it was his time to go.

In the month of June when I had those pains, I went to the Emergency Room and the doctor told me I required the surgery, I almost broke down. My first thoughts were 'why couldn't this have happened before John died so that I could have some support?'

As I thought about it, I decided to contact the Organ Procurement Organization and I asked if any of John's bone was available. Because by the time the final donation and the decision had been made to have surgery took place, it was already August. John had died three months earlier and I figured the tissue was already gone.

Unbeknownst to me there is a long process of preparing the tissue and his bone was right at the point where they give it the final treatment which will determine what the bone can be used for. And so they made sure that his bone was prepared so that I could receive a piece of his bone as a graft

I waited an extra couple of months. I didn't have the surgery until October because I decided to wait until his bone was to be available.

I received my transplant and I had not realized that I had actually lost strength in my left arm. I am right-handed and I don't really use my left arm for much.

I realized after the fact that what I thought was being a butter-finger, you know, 'oops, I dropped that.' It wasn't that it was just slipping out of my hand; my hand did not have the strength to hold things.

After I was diagnosed, I began to notice. Picking up a quart of milk made my arm tremble. It was the maximum weight I was capable of holding.

After the surgery, not only did I become renewed, I have total use of my arm. I have no pain in the arm. As a matter of fact, six weeks post surgery the bone was partially absorbed.

So I just want to thank you for your great gifts. I know that each gift is a sacrifice and I want to thank you for making that choice.

By Jean Reyes de Gonzalez
(Transcript of speech given at the National Donor Recognition Ceremony, July 25, 2005.)
Reprinted By Permission

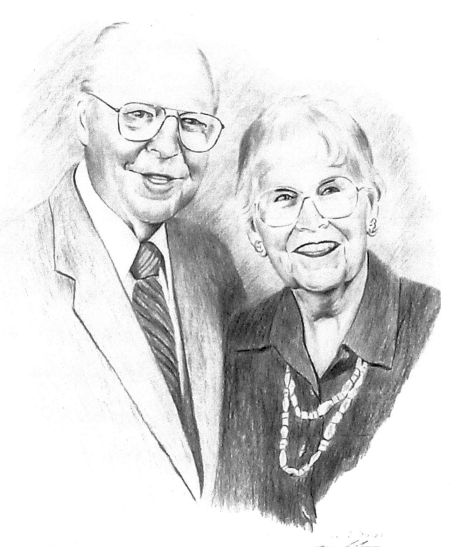

Bill and Marge Falsey

29

I Never Asked The Question

As I sat with my Father on the front porch of my Kansas City home, I could see that things were somehow different. I couldn't quite put my finger on it, but there was definitely a difference in my Father. Normally an active person, always doing something, Dad seemed content on this particular day just sitting on the front porch watching the world go by. He was deep in thought about something – but what?

The porch was not the old-fashioned type designed for visiting. No, it was the modern type, with barely enough room for two people to stand. Yet, we each sat in lawn chairs blocking the screen door, not allowing anyone else to come or go.

Dad was tired from a long drive. He and Mom had just driven from Phoenix, Arizona, stopping in Kansas City on their way to Holland, Michigan. Mom and Dad were both in their 80s, and we children were not comfortable with them driving so far, but they would hear nothing of it. They had made the journey many times before, and they wanted to make it one more time.

There was a time not so long ago when they would commute between the two states, from their summer home in Michigan to their winter home in Arizona and back again as the seasons changed. That is one reason my wife, Joyce, and I chose to live in Kansas City. Being about halfway along the route ensured that we would see them as they made the semi-annual journey.

The trip became too much for them a few years back, so they sold the house in Michigan and became permanent residents of Arizona. But years had passed and they wanted to make the journey one more time.

As we sat there, Dad asked questions about my upcoming surgery. I was scheduled to donate a kidney to my nephew Aaron in a few weeks, and Dad was the curious type who wanted to know about everything. In his lifetime, organ transplantation had grown from a dream, to an experiment, to an almost-everyday occurrence. He wanted to know more.

He had far more questions than I could answer. All I knew was that I was a match for Aaron and, since Aaron needed my kidney, it seemed only right to give it to him.

Aaron, my wife's brother's son, and I were not biologically related. That fact was the primary reason I decided to give him my kidney. When we matched four of six antigens, it was the only logical thing to do. I didn't know much about what constitutes a match, but I did know that matching four of six is a better match than a brother would be expected to be.

I look at things in simplistic terms. There are six numbers on a lottery ticket and it's very rare to match four. Matching Aaron so well just showed me it was meant to be, and I never gave it much thought. God was telling me something, and I was not about to ignore Him.

As Dad asked more and more questions about my upcoming surgery, I grew uncomfortable. He wanted to know so many details, details I did not have. I knew enough about surgery that I didn't want too many details.

I didn't want to know how much it would hurt, or dwell on the risks. I chose instead to trust in God and leave the details in His hands. Like matching the numbers on the lottery ticket, I felt this was destiny.

My sister-in-law, Joan, had already donated a kidney to Aaron several years ago. I had seen her recover from the surgery and figured I would do the same.

I knew it was very painful for her, but she soon forgot about the pain when she saw the change it made in her son. Women have a way of doing that. They give birth, but soon enough, they forget about the pain and remember only the joy of giving life.

Joan's kidney worked right away and Aaron began to feel better immediately. As soon as Aaron was able to walk after surgery, he walked to his Mother's room to thank her.

Okay, maybe she wanted to slap him just once when he walked into her hospital room all healthy and happy. She was in pain and unable to move, and he was already up and walking. She wanted it that way, of course, but what would one slap on the cheek hurt?

Joan's momentary pain was replaced with a permanent joy. She had given her son life at birth and then had another opportunity to renew his life years later.

I had never had surgery before; I couldn't know how much it would hurt. When Joan tried to talk about her experience, I just tuned her out. I figured it would be bad enough, but there was no point in dwelling on it. She had survived it and forgotten about the pain. I could survive and forget about the pain too.

Now her transplanted kidney was failing in Aaron and he needed a replacement. If I were compatible, I wanted to be his donor. And it seemed like I was compatible.

My Father wondered aloud if anyone would want his organs. He was 85 and reasonably healthy, but there is a limit to how long the body lasts. He was closer to the end of life than the beginning and didn't know if his organs had enough life left. Would anyone want his organs when he died? It was a question that eventually would haunt me.

Our visit drew to a close too quickly. Mom and Dad left the next morning to continue their cross-country journey. We expected to see each other again soon; Mom and Dad planned to travel to Omaha to be with me during my recovery.

Worried about their long drive, we called Mom and Dad at each stop along the way. Each time we were relieved to hear of their progress and how much fun they were having visiting friends and family. All but one of their children lived along the route. This was a good excuse to visit them all and slow down the pace of the trip.

When the trip was over and they were safely back in Arizona, my Father called all of us to let us know they had made it back home.

I still remember the defiant message he left on our answering machine: "We made it home, so you can stop worrying about us." It was great news, because he had recognized that we were worried, and because he still had his sense of humor.

My attention turned back to the impending kidney

donation and all the preparation for being out of town for a few weeks. We didn't know how long we would be in Omaha, but knew we would be there for a while. All we needed was one final cross-match result and we would be on our way. The cross-match would tell us if the transplant would likely be successful.

With everything packed, we waited for a phone call with the test results. There was every reason to believe we would be on the road soon. I thought the final cross-match was nothing more than a formality. I was wrong.

Less than two days before the scheduled surgery, we learned that Aaron and I had a positive cross-match, which meant that the kidney most likely would be rejected. Our travel plans were suddenly put on hold. As soon as I heard the news, I called my parents. They would have to cancel their trip, too.

My Father was one to always put a positive spin on things. Knowing I was disappointed about the surgery, he wanted to cheer me up. He mentioned that he had so many people praying for me, that I would be pretty safe for a while.

I asked, "You mean I could go play in traffic if I wanted to?"

"Yeah, you probably could," he responded.

* * *

On June 1, exactly one week after the transplant was scheduled to take place; Joyce and I were just about to go to bed. It was early for a Friday night, but we were tired from the exhausting weeks we had gone through. For the first time in months, we had no plans and that meant an opportunity to catch up on much-needed sleep. Shortly before 10 o'clock, the phone rang. Because it's later than we normally get calls, we both just assumed it was a wrong number. Instead, my older sister, Kathie, was on the line. She had barely said hello when her voice cracked. Something was wrong, very wrong. There was no small talk; she got directly to the point. "Mom and Dad were in an accident…"

"Are they okay?" I asked, assuming that they were.

There was a pause that seemed to last an eternity. Her voice cracked even more and her voice got much softer when she replied, "Mom was killed instantly."

"Oh, my God. What about Dad? How is he taking it? How is he? Is he okay?" I wondered.

"He was alive but unconscious when the paramedics arrived … but there was nothing they could do. He died there at the scene," she said.

With that very brief conversation, my life had changed. My Mom and my Dad were dead.

Kathie and I talked for quite a while trying to figure out what we could do. Trying to figure out what had happened. There were few details available, but the brutal truth was that Mom and Dad had died suddenly on an Arizona highway only about five miles from their home. They had recently traveled 5,000 miles across the country without incident and then, five miles from home, a tractor-trailer crossed over into their lane and hit them head-on.

Among the details known, there were a few that brought us some comfort. The accident was so brutal that there was absolutely no way my parents could have suffered. They had died without knowing what had hit them. They were traveling 60 miles an hour in one direction and then, a second later, were traveling backward.

The incredible force was too much for any human being to absorb – let alone a pair of frail octogenarians. They could not have suffered – it simply was not possible.

I had many more questions than Kathie could answer. No one could answer all of the inevitable questions, especially so early after the fact. We could only imagine and speculate on the few facts known, and hope for the best on the unknown.

How ironic it was that we worried about *their* driving and they died in an automobile accident through no fault of their own. And the last words my Father and I exchanged were about prayer and traffic. Mom and Dad died in traffic, and we now could do nothing for them but pray.

I remembered my Father wondering aloud just six weeks earlier if anyone would be able to use his organs when he died. I could not have imagined that we would have to find the answer to his question so soon.

What would he have wanted?

All of us wanted to honor his wishes, but we didn't know his wishes. What if they asked us about donating his organs? What would be the right thing to do?

We didn't know Mom's wishes either. It was too late to ask either one of them, yet we could be asked to make a critical decision.

What if we made the wrong choice?

Those were all questions running through my mind, and I simply didn't know the answers.

As much as I worried about not being able to adequately respond to those questions, we soon learned the answer didn't really matter. Mom and Dad were not candidates for organ transplantation. Age, medication and other factors ruled them out. They might have been candidates for bone or tissue donation, but we will never know because we were not asked about those possibilities.

As I look back, it is somewhat surprising that neither Mom nor Dad expressed their feelings about being organ donors. They were very careful to make their feelings known about so many things.

I remember my Mom once asking the question, "If something were to happen to us in Arizona, would you mind if we had a small ceremony here and were cremated and buried in Michigan?" It was a simple question, but in that one question Mom let us know what she and Dad wanted done with their bodies after they finished using them. It was a simple request that was easy to carry out, but only because Mom let us know what she and Dad wanted.

Those were things we could do. And yes, we did those things precisely because we knew what they wanted. It was comforting to do such a little thing for them now.

Time has passed and, now that the fog of the accident has cleared, I no longer wonder what my parents would have wanted if they had been candidates for organ donation. They were incredibly giving people who gave more to charity than anyone could have expected. Of course, I now know what they would have wanted. At the time of the accident though? No, I didn't know; none of us did. It would have been a tragic mistake to take the easy road and say, "No."

Epilogue

If I had to offer advice for anyone considering becoming an organ donor, it would be this – carefully think about what you want, and let others know how you feel. Whether your desire is to be an organ donor after death, or a living organ donor, you shouldn't go down this path alone. Support from friends and family is important.

If you want to become a donor upon your death, the most important thing is to let your family know. Signing your driver's license is good advice, as is joining your state organ donor registry. In the end however, it may not be enough. In some states, it is the family of the deceased that makes the ultimate decision. And the family cannot honor wishes without being aware of those wishes. At that tragic time, it is simply too late to ask.

There is another benefit about talking with your family about donation. You may be called upon to make a decision for someone you love. It is a tough decision, but far easier if you know what the person would have wanted. And it will be comforting to know you honored their wishes.

If you are considering becoming a living donor, it is also important to discuss it with your family. Organ donation is major surgery and there are risks. Whether the surgery goes perfectly or there are major problems, you will need the help of others. If you have a good support system from family or friends, you will be far better off. The risks you are taking affect others as well.

Perhaps the best advice is to do your homework. Contact other donors and ask for their guidance, and listen to their experience. An outstanding web-site to meet donors is Living Donors Online (www.living-donorsonline.org). It is a web-site by organ donors, for organ donors. Topics are wide open on the discussion board and posters will discuss almost anything. This is the site where Karol (chapter 21) found a donor for her daughter (chapter 22).

The choice of a transplant center may be a difficult one. The Scientific Registry of Transplant Recipients (SRTR) covers a full range of transplant activities in the United States on their web-site www.ustrans-plant.org. Included in the statistics is center specific data that allows the reader to compare the experience and track records of transplant centers.

The Living Organ Donor Advocacy Program, www.lodap.com provides a wealth of knowledge for those considering becoming donors. Founded in 2001 by Kimberly Tracy, a nurse and a kidney donor, this site promotes efforts to insure the safety of living organ donors. Included on the site are helpful hints of what to do before donating an organ, and how to obtain help for those who have experienced problems.

The National Kidney Foundation (www.kidney.org) and the United Network of Organ Sharing (www.uons.org and transplantliving.org) also have web-sites packed with information about transplanta-tion.

If you cannot find answers to specific questions, do not be afraid to ask. There are no stupid questions. Each year more than 25,000 patients receive trans-plants, and more than 6,000 of the organs come from living donors. Many, if not most, are anxious to talk about their experiences.

Although there is little data on the long term outcome of living organ donors, most donors appear to do very well. Advocates continue to push for a living organ donor registry, but at present, the national registry doesn't exist. The Living Organ Donor Network (LODN) tracks some living kidney donors and offers insurance protection for complications following kidney donation. Information about this important program can be obtained from the South Eastern Organ Procurement Foundation www.seopf.org.

There is little doubt that organ transplantation enhances the lives of recipients, and is cost effective too. About three quarters of the people on the wait list are waiting for kidneys, and it is estimated that each kidney transplant saves Medicare between $250,000 and $970,000. Without a transplant, candidates require dialysis which is paid primarily by Medicare.

Organ Donation & Religion

Does Your Religion Support Organ Donation?

Although there are variations, most major religions support or permit organ donation. Following is a listing of religions and their view of organ donation from the National Kidney Foundation web-site www.kidney.org. This is reprinted by permission of the National Kidney Foundation.

AME & AME ZION (African Methodist Episcopal)

Donation is viewed as an act of neighborly love and charity by these denominations. They encourage all members to support donation as a way of helping others.

Amish

The Amish approve of transplantation if there is a definite indication that the health of the recipient would improve.

Assembly Of God

The Church has no official policy in regards to donation. The decision to donate is left up to the individual. Donation is highly supported by the denomination.

Baptist

Donation is supported as an act of charity and the church leaves the decision to donate up to the individual.

Brethren

The Church of the Brethren's Annual Conference in 1993 wrote a resolution on organ and tissue donation in support and encouragement of donation. They wrote that, "We have the opportunity to help others out of love for Christ, through the donation of organs and tissues."

Buddhism

Buddhists believe that donation is a matter of individual conscience and place high value on acts of compassion. They emphasize the importance of letting family members know one's wishes as relates to Donation.

Catholicism

Transplants are acceptable to the Vatican and donation is encouraged as an act of charity and love.

Christian Church (Disciples of Christ)

The Christian Church encourages donation. They believe that humans were created for God's glory and for sharing God's love.

Christian Science

Christian scientists do not maintain a position on donation, leaving it to the individual to decide.

Episcopal

The Episcopal Church passed a resolution in 1982 that recognizes the life-giving benefits of organ, blood, and tissue donation. All Christians are encouraged to become organ, blood, and tissue donors "as part of their ministry to others in the name of Christ, who gave His life that we may have life in its fullness."

Greek Orthodox

The Greek Orthodox Church has no objection to donation as long as the organs and tissues are used to better human life.

Gypsies

Gypsies are a people of different ethnic groups without a formalized religion. They share common folk beliefs and tend to be opposed to donation. Their opposition is connected with their beliefs about the afterlife. Traditional belief contends that for one year after death, the soul retraces its steps. Thus, the body must remain intact because the soul maintains its physical shape.

Hinduism
Donation of organs is an individual decision and is not against the Hindu religion.

Independent Conservative Evangelical
Generally, Evangelicals have no opposition to donation. Each church is autonomous and leaves the decision to donate up to the individual.

Islam
The religion of Islam strongly believes in the principle of saving human lives. According to A. Sachedina in his Transplantation Proceedings' article, Islamic Views on organ transplantation, "the majority of the Muslim scholars belonging to various schools of Islamic law have invoked the principle of priority of saving human life and have permitted the organ transplant as a necessity to procure that noble end."

Jehovah's Witnesses
Donation is a matter of individual conscience with provision that all organs and tissues be completely drained of blood.

Judaism
Jews believe that if it is possible to donate an organ to save a life, it is obligatory to do so. Since restoring sight is considered life saving, this includes cornea organ transplantation.

Lutheran
In 1984, the Lutheran Church in America passed a resolution stating that donation contributes to the well-being of humanity and can be "an expression of sacrificial love for a neighbor in need." They call on "members to consider donating organs and to make any necessary family and legal arrangements, including the use of a signed donor card."

Mennonite
Mennonites have no formal position on donation, but are not

opposed to it. They believe the decision to donate is up to the individual and/or their family.

Mormon (Church of Jesus Christ of Latter-Day Saints)

The Church of Jesus Christ of Latter-Day Saints believes that the decision to donate is an individual one made in conjunction with family, medical personnel, and prayer. They do not oppose donation.

Pentecostal

Pentecostals believe that the decision to donate should be left up to the individual.

Presbyterian

Presbyterians encourage and support donation. They respect a person's right to make decisions regarding their own body.

Protestantism

Encourage and endorse Donation.

Seventh-Day Adventist

Donation and transplantation are strongly encouraged by Seventh-Day Adventists. They have many transplant hospitals, including Loma Linda in California. Loma Linda specializes in pediatric heart transplantation.

Shinto

In Shinto, the dead body is considered to be impure and dangerous, and thus quite powerful. "In folk belief context, injuring a dead body is a serious crime. . .", according to E. Narnihira in his article, "Shinto Concept Concerning the Dead Hutnan Body." "To this day it is difficult to obtain consent from bereaved families for donation or dissection for medical education or pathological anatomy . . . the Japanese regards them all in the sense of injuring a dead body." Families are concerned that they not injure the itai - the relationship between the dead person and the bereaved people.

Society of Friends (Quakers)

Donation is believed to be an individual decision. The Society of Friends does not have an official position on donation.

Unitarian Universalists

Donation is widely supported by Unitarian Universalists. They view it as an act of love and selfless giving.

United Church of Christ

The United Church of Christ supports and encourages donation.

United Methodist

The United Methodist Church issued a policy statement in regards to donation. In it, they state that "The United Methodist Church recognizes the life-giving benefits of donation, and thereby encourages all Christians to become donors by signing and carrying cards or driver's licenses, attesting to their commitment of such organs upon their death, to those in need, as a part of their ministry to others in the name of Christ, who gave His life that we might have life in its fullness."

About the
Artist

James A Jackson Jr. has a real zeal for life. "I've done a lot of things in my life and I'm not done yet. I just like to try different things." His curiosity and diverse interests are reflected in his art. James works with a number of mediums including oil paintings, water colors and pencil sketching. Even when relaxing on a summer day, you may find James honing his artistic talents with his 'solar etchings' – burning images into wood using only a magnifying glass and the power of the sun.

Although he is characteristically private and shy, he has always had big plans and dreams. Now that he has retired from the corporate life, he is concentrating on his art. He runs a business, Special Occasion Portraits, selling original pieces as well as commissioned portraits. He has drawn historical figures such as General Colin Powell and General Benjamin O. Davis Jr., Commander of the Tuskegee Airmen.

James' pencil sketches appear throughout this book.

Special Occasion Portraits
P. O. Box 860
Winfield, KS 67156
www.specialoccasionportraits.com
email: jjgifting@yahoo.com

About the
Author

Tom Falsey has a passion for organ donor awareness and his passion is backed up with action. Tom was the first anonymous kidney donor at The Nebraska Medical Center, and he is one of five kidney donors in his extended family. Tom has also been on the bone marrow registry for over fifteen years and has donated more than 75 units of blood components.

Tom Falsey has served on numerous boards and committees involved in organ donation including: United Network of Organ Sharing (UNOS) Board of Directors (2005 – 2008), Organ Procurement and Transplantation Network (OPTN) Board of Directors (2005 – 2008), National Kidney Foundation (NKF) of Kansas and Western Missouri Board of Directors (2007), UNOS Living Donor Committee (2006 – 2008), and UNOS Nominating Committee (2007).

Mr. Falsey has been widely quoted in local and national media including; Wall Street Journal, USA Today, CBS Early Show, People magazine and the National Examiner.

**Additional copies of this book are available
directly from the publisher**

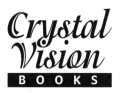

P.O. Box 3185
Shawnee, Kansas 66216

Special discounts are available for Transplant Centers
and Organ Procurement Organizations.